PRIMER OF
EPIDEMIOLOGY

PRIMER OF EPIDEMIOLOGY

Gary D. Friedman

M.D., S.M. in Hyg., F.A.C.P.

Senior Epidemiologist, Department of Medical Methods Research, Kaiser-Permanente Medical Care Program

Assistant Clinical Professor of Medicine and of Ambulatory and Community Medicine, University of California School of Medicine, San Francisco

Lecturer in Epidemiology, University of California School of Public Health, Berkeley

McGRAW-HILL BOOK COMPANY

A Blakiston Publication

New York St. Louis San Francisco Düsseldorf Johannesburg
Kuala Lumpur London Mexico Montreal New Delhi Panama
Paris São Paulo Singapore Sydney Tokyo Toronto

**PRIMER OF
EPIDEMIOLOGY**

7890MUMU7987

This book was set in Helvetica by Black Dot, Inc. The editors were
Paul K. Schneider and Shelly Levine Langman; the designer was
Joseph Gillians; and the production supervisor was
Thomas J. LoPinto. The drawings were done
by Eric G. Hieber Associates Inc.
The Murray Printing Company was printer and binder.

Library of Congress Cataloging in Publication Data

Friedman, Gary D   date
    Primer of epidemiology.

    "A Blakiston publication."
    1. Epidemiology. I. Title. [DNLM: 1. Epidemi-
ology. WA100 F911p 1974]
RA651.F68   614.4   73-20037
ISBN 0-07-022425-0

To Ruth,
Emily,
Justin,
and Richard

CONTENTS

PREFACE

It has seemed to me that many health-care professionals do not have an adequate understanding or appreciation of what epidemiology is all about or how it relates to their own work. Furthermore, one frequently finds a failure in communication between the clinician and the epidemiologist despite their common concern over human health and disease. I believe it is fair to say that most students of medicine and other health sciences regard epidemiology as a boring and irrelevant subject which they study only because they are required to. Another common view of epidemiology among health-care professionals is that it is highly esoteric or mathematical and too complex for them to understand.

With those problems in mind I have attempted to write a concise textbook for physicians, medical students, and other health-care professionals that would explain epidemiologic concepts clearly and simply. I have also tried to bridge the gap in communication between the clinician and epidemiologist in a variety of ways, such as providing a number of clinical examples throughout the book, explaining to the clinician why the epidemiologic emphasis on the study of groups rather than individuals is necessary, and trying to show the relevance of epidemiology to the major concerns of the clinician such as diagnosis and choice of therapy. Also, I have described several interesting epidemiologic studies to illustrate various methods of investigation. Rather than showing just tables of data to illustrate the results of these studies, I have tried to describe them in sufficient detail so the reader will come away with a real feeling for what it is like to carry out an epidemiologic study. I have attempted, also, to provide some much sought-after practical advice on how to conduct a simple epidemiologic or clinical study and on critical reading of the medical literature. Finally, there is some discussion of epidemiology in relation to the study of problems currently of great social and political importance—the changing health care system and environmental hazards.

Some epidemiologists may be disappointed at the lack of discussion of some of the epidemiologic classics such as Snow's studies of cholera or Goldberger's studies of pellagra. Despite the importance and beauty of these studies, I believe that most students are much more interested in examples that relate to current health and social problems.

Few, if any, of the ideas and concepts in this book are original. I am deeply indebted to those who trained me in epidemiology and related subjects and to the many colleagues and friends with whom I have worked over the past decade for all I have learned from them. A number of the examples, references, and other materials that appear here were suggested to me by colleagues, to whom I am most grateful. It would be impossible for me to name all who, in one way or another, helped me to write this book, but I hope they are aware of my appreciation.

I would like to single out for special thanks Dr. Loring G. Dales, Dr. Mark J. Yanover, and my wife, Ruth, who read the entire manuscript carefully during its preparation and made many valuable suggestions. I am grateful to Mrs. Agnes M. Lewis for carefully typing the manuscript and drawing some of the figures, and to Dr. Morris F. Collen for his advice and encouragement.

Gary D. Friedman

Chapter 1

Introduction to Epidemiology

EPIDEMIOLOGY: DEFINITION, PURPOSE, AND RELATION TO PATIENT CARE

Epidemiology is the study of disease occurrence in human populations. The primary units of concern are *groups* of persons, not separate individuals. Thinking in epidemiologic terms often seems foreign to clinicians and other health-care professionals, who are trained to think of the unique problems of each particular patient.

Whether one focuses on individuals or groups should depend upon what one is trying to accomplish. In caring for a sick patient, the need to individualize the diagnosis and treatment for that unique patient is obvious. However, groups of persons must be studied in order to answer certain important questions. These questions often relate to the etiology and prevention of disease and to the allocation of effort and resources in health-care facilities and in communities.

Some examples of questions that require epidemiologic study of human populations are:

When can we expect the next influenza epidemic?
Why are we seeing so much coronary heart disease these days?
How can cancer of the uterine cervix best be prevented?
How often should healthy patients be given medical checkups and what examinations and tests should these checkups include?

Although they also focus on groups, clinical studies of the natural course of disease or the effects of treatments should be distinguished from epidemiologic studies. In general, epidemiologists are more concerned with disease patterns in natural populations such as communities or nations. Clinical studies, on the other hand, are concerned with groups of *patients* seen in a medical facility. However, the methods of investigation are often quite similar, so that training and experience in epidemiology are useful for the clinical investigator.

In addition to being related to clinical research, epidemiology is intimately involved in clinical practice. Clinicians regularly use epidemiologic knowledge in the diagnosis and treatment of disease. Accordingly, after the elements of epidemiology are presented in subsequent chapters, the relationship of epidemiology to clinical research and to medical care will be described.

How Epidemiology Contributes to Understanding Disease Etiology

Each scientific discipline in medicine is uniquely able to answer certain questions. If our goal is to understand how a particular disease occurs, each discipline can attack the problem at its own level and contribute to our understanding.

It is sometimes implied that the purpose of epidemiology is to provide clues to etiology which can later assist the laboratory scientist in arriving at the real answer. This is a distorted view. There are certain questions that can only be answered outside of the laboratory.

A new vaccine may be developed and prepared by biologists

and biochemists, but epidemiologists will have to answer whether the vaccine is successful in preventing disease.

Similarly, laboratory scientists can identify carcinogenic compounds in tobacco smoke and may even be able to produce lung cancer in experimental animals by forcing them to smoke cigarettes. However, the idea that cigarette smoking causes human lung cancer would be unconvincing unless epidemiologists also showed that lung cancer occurred more often in cigarette smokers than in nonsmokers.

Causation of Disease A moment's thought about any disease reveals that more than one factor contributes to its occurrence. For example, tuberculosis is not merely caused by the tubercle bacillus. Not everyone exposed to the tubercle bacillus becomes ill with tuberculosis. Other factors have been identified which clearly contribute to the occurrence of this disease. These factors include poverty, overcrowding, malnutrition, and alcoholism. Amelioration of these other factors can do much to prevent this disease.

Epidemiologists have organized the complex multifactorial process that leads to disease in various ways. One useful way to view the causation of some diseases, particularly certain infectious diseases, is in tripartite terms of the agent, the environment, and the host. For acute rheumatic fever the agent is the beta-hemolytic streptococcus. However, not all persons infected with this organism develop the disease. Thus, considerations of host susceptibility are important. Constitutional factors appear to play a role not only in whether or not the disease develops but also in the localization of cardiac damage. Important environmental factors include social conditions such as poverty and crowding as well as nonhuman aspects of the environment such as season, climate, and altitude.

Another epidemiologic view of disease etiology is as a "web of causation." This concept of disease causation considers all the predisposing factors of any type and their complex relations with each other and with the disease. One current view of the multiple factors leading to myocardial infarction well illustrates a causal web (Fig. 1-1). (Despite the apparent complexity of this diagram, it is undoubtedly an oversimplification and will certainly be modified by further study.) Note that many interrelated factors ultimately lead to

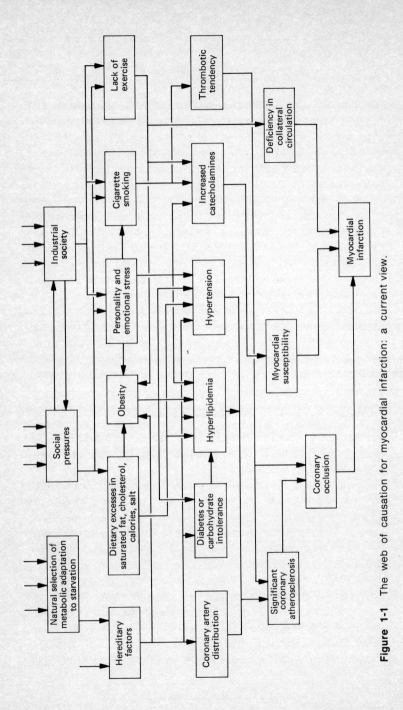

Figure 1-1 The web of causation for myocardial infarction: a current view.

myocardial infarction. Each of these factors mentioned is also influenced by a variety of other factors not shown, leading to as complex a causal web as one chooses to construct. Nevertheless, based on the information presented, it can be seen that a variety of actions could be taken which might reduce the occurrence of myocardial infarction. These actions include dietary modifications, treatment of hypertension, and changing public attitudes toward smoking and exercise.

It is tempting to search for a primary cause, or the most important or most direct of the many causal factors. The benefits of this search are perhaps more philosophical or psychological than practical. In terms of disease prevention it may be most practical to attack a causal web at a spot that seems relatively remote from the disease. To prevent malaria, we do not merely try to destroy the malaria parasite; rather, we drain swamps to control the mosquito population, since this is a practical and effective approach. Similarly, economic development and general improvements in living conditions seem to have done more to reduce mortality from tuberculosis than any chemotherapeutic agent directed specifically at the tubercle bacillus.

Definition and Classification of Diseases

No discussion of disease causation would be complete without some comment about the relatively arbitrary and varying ways in which diseases are defined.

What physicians are faced with are ill persons! However, it has been convenient and valuable to divide the ill persons into categories and give each category a name. We call each category a disease. Ill people do not always fit well into our categories, as any physician will discover if he tries to practice medicine using only the textbooks.

We name diseases to reflect something about our perception or understanding of what the disease entails. Some disease names are merely descriptive of some aspect such as appearance (e.g., erythema multiforme) or subjective sensation (e.g., headache). Some names probe a bit deeper but are still descriptive of pathologic anatomy, often as defined by gross or microscopic appearance (e.g., adenocarcinoma of the colon or fracture of the femur). On the other hand, the disease name may focus on some real or supposed causative factor; e.g., pneumococcal pneumonia implies a pulmonary infection by the pneumococcus.

As knowledge about disease causation increases, the disease names are often switched from descriptive terms to terms implying a causal factor. Many ill persons who had been formerly named by a variety of descriptive terms become reclassified under a single causal heading. Similarly, a single descriptive heading may have contained patients with a variety of causally defined diseases. One of the former names for the condition we now call tuberculosis was *phthisis*, meaning "wasting away." Patients in whom wasting dominates the clinical picture constitute only a portion of persons with tuberculosis, and tuberculosis is only one of the causes of wasting.

Causal names for disease are useful in that they immediately imply means for prevention or therapy; in fact, they can drastically change the manner in which a particular health problem is handled. However, causal names can also lead to problems. When the focus on one causal factor such as an infectious agent is reflected in the disease name, we often forget that other factors are operating and tend to regard the infectious or other agent as the only cause.

In summary, disease names are important tools for thought and communication. However they must be viewed in proper perspective. They tend to mask differences among patients, and they have a way of influencing and narrowing our thinking. Disease names may even become "the thing itself," whereas the emphasis should be on the ill person. Furthermore, disease names are transitory. The naming and classifying of ill persons has changed markedly through history and will continue to change.

REFERENCE

MacMahon, B., and T. F. Pugh, *Epidemiology: Principles and Methods.* (Boston: Little, Brown, 1970), Chaps. 1, 2, and 4.

Chapter 2

Basic Measurements in Epidemiology

There is one thing I would be glad to ask you. When a mathematician engaged in investigating physical actions and results has arrived at his conclusions, may they not be expressed in common language as fully, clearly, and definitely as in mathematical formulae? If so, would it not be a great boon to such as I to express them so?

Michael Faraday,
Letter to James Clerk Maxwell

Epidemiology is a quantitative science. Its measured quantities and descriptive terms are used to describe *groups* of persons.

Counts The simplest and most frequently performed quantitative measurement in epidemiology is a count of the number of persons in the group studied who have a particular disease or a particular characteristic. For example, it may be noted that 10 people in a college dormitory developed infectious hepatitis or that 16 stomach cancer patients were foreign-born.

Proportions and Rates

In order for a count to be descriptive of a group it must be seen in proportion to it; i.e., it must be divided by the total number in the group. The 10 hepatitis cases would have quite a different significance for the dormitory if the dormitory housed 500 students than if it housed only 20. In the first case the proportion would be $^{10}/_{500}$, or 0.02, or 2 percent. (Percentage, or number per one hundred, is one of the most common ways of expressing proportions. Number per 1,000 or 1 million, or any other convenient base may be used.) In the second case the proportion would be $^{10}/_{20}$ or 0.50.

The use of denominators to convert counts into proportions seems almost too simple to mention. However, a proportion is one basic way to describe a group. *One of the central concerns of epidemiology is to find and enumerate appropriate denominators in order to describe and to compare groups in a meaningful and useful way.*

Certain kinds of proportions are used very frequently in epidemiology. These are referred to as *rates.* The various types of rates involve or imply some time relationship. The two most commonly used rates which every physician should understand and remember are the prevalence rate and the incidence rate:

Prevalence Rate

$$\text{Prevalence rate} = \frac{\text{number of persons with a disease}}{\text{total number in group}}$$

Prevalence describes a group at a certain point in time. It is like a snapshot of an existing situation. For example, *the prevalence of electrocardiographic abnormalities at our screening examination was 5 percent*; or, *the prevalence of diarrhea in the children's camp on July 13 was 33 percent.* Or, *the prevalence of significant hyperbilirubinemia in full-term infants on the third postpartum day is 20 percent.* As can be seen by the above examples the point in time is not necessarily a true geometric point with no length, but is a relatively short time such as a day. Nor does the point have to be in calendar time. It can refer to an event which may happen to different persons at different times, such as an examination or the third postpartum day.

Incidence Rate

$$\text{Incidence rate} = \frac{\text{number of persons developing a disease}}{\text{total number at risk}} \text{ per unit of time}$$

Incidence describes the rate of development of a disease in a group over a period of time, which is included in the denominator. In contrast to a snapshot, incidence describes a continuing process over a given time period. For example, *the incidence of myocardial infarction is about 1 percent per year in men aged 55–59 in our community*; or, *at the height of the epidemic the incidence of chicken pox in the first grade children was 10 percent per day.*

Not everyone in a study population may be at risk for developing a disease. For example, some diseases are lifelong in duration, so that once you have it you cannot develop it again. Persons with such a disease are usually removed from the denominator population at risk.

In the medical literature the word "incidence" is often used to describe prevalence or simple proportion. For example, *the incidence of gallstones is 20 percent in middle-aged women*; or, *in our autopsy series the incidence of liver cirrhosis was 12 percent.* This imprecise use of "incidence" should be avoided, since the specific concept of incidence, defined as a rate of development, is a useful one.

Other Rates Some other rates, often used in epidemiology, are described below.

$$\text{Period prevalence} = \frac{\text{number of persons with a disease during a period of time}}{\text{total number in group}}$$

Sometimes one wishes to have a measure of all the diseases affecting a group during a period of time such as the year, 1970, rather than at a point in time. The period prevalence of a disease in 1970 turns out to be the prevalence at the beginning of 1970 plus the annual incidence during 1970.

Mortality, or death, rate =
$$\frac{\text{number of persons dying (due to a particular cause or due to all causes)}}{\text{total number in group}} \text{ per unit of time}$$

Mortality rate is analogous to incidence but refers to the process of dying rather than the process of becoming ill.

Any rate may refer to a subgroup of a population. For example:

Age–specific mortality rate =
$$\frac{\text{number of persons dying in a particular age group}}{\text{total number in the same age group}} \text{ per unit of time}$$

$$\text{Case fatality rate} = \frac{\text{number of persons dying due to a particular disease}}{\text{total number with the disease}}$$

Case fatality rate refers to the proportion of persons with a particular disease who die. The time element is usually not specified but may be, if desired, as with incidence.

A variety of other disease rates are described by Siegel (1967). In most rates the numerator must include only persons who are derived from the denominator population. The denominator is considered the total population at risk of being or becoming one of the numerator. Thus, these rates can be viewed as a statement of probability that a condition exists (prevalence) or will develop (incidence) in the population at risk.

Some rates depart somewhat from the ideal of having the numerator being derived from the denominator population at risk. This is done for convenience, because of the ready availability of data that approximate the ideal. Consider the

Maternal mortality rate =

number of deaths from puerperal causes during a year

number of live births during the same year

Actually, the true population of mothers at risk for puerperal death includes those that have had stillbirths as well as those that have had live births. Legally required registration and counting of live births makes this live-birth denominator much more accessible.

Handling Changing Denominators If a denominator population is growing or shrinking during the period of time for which a rate is to be computed, then it is customary to use the population size at the *midpoint* of the time interval as an estimate of the average population at risk. If an incidence rate is to be computed for the year 1973, then the population at risk as of July 1, 1973 is used for the denominator.

Comparison of Rates, Using Differences or Ratios

Differences It is often desired to compare a rate in one group with that in another. One may simply note both rates and observe that one is larger than the other. By subtracting the smaller from the larger, one may obtain the magnitude of the difference.

The difference between two incidence rates is sometimes called "attributable risk" if the two groups being compared differ in some other aspect that is believed to play a causal role in the disease. For example, in Hammond's (1966) study of smoking and mortality the lung cancer mortality rate in nonsmokers ages 55–69 was 19 per 100,000 persons per year as compared to 188 per 100,000 in cigarette smokers. The difference between the two lung cancer mortality rates was 169 per 100,000 per year. This is the lung cancer risk attributable to smoking, *if* smoking is the only important difference between the groups in factors affecting the development of lung cancer. Only the *excess* rate in smokers should be attributed to smoking—not the entire smokers' incidence rate—since non-smokers develop some lung cancer, too.

Ratios Another way to compare two rates is by determining the ratio of one to the other, that is, dividing one by the other. In the smoking and lung cancer example, the ratio of the rate in smokers to that in nonsmokers was $^{188}/_{19}$ or 9.9. The smokers had a 9.9 times greater risk of dying from lung cancer than did the nonsmokers. The ratio of two rates is sometimes called the "relative risk," "risk ratio," "morbidity ratio," or, if mortality rates are under consideration, the "mortality ratio."

Ratio Comparisons of Several Groups to a Single Standard
When one wishes to compare several different rates, it is often convenient to determine the ratio of all the different rates to a single standard. The standard of comparison may be an actual rate for a particular group that seems appropriate to use. In the study of smoking and lung cancer, smokers were divided according to the number of cigarettes currently smoked per day. Nonsmokers were again used as the standard of comparison, and their mortality rate was arbitrarily designated as 1.0. In comparison, the ratios for male smokers, ages 55–69, were 3.5 for smokers of 1 to 9 cigarettes per day, 8.8 for smokers of 10 to 19 cigarettes per day, 13.8 for smokers of 20 to 39 cigarettes per day, and 17.5 for smokers of 40 or more cigarettes per day.

It may be that the group to be used as a standard differs from the other groups in some important respect, resulting in a biased or unfair comparison. For example, suppose that the men in the different smoking categories not only had different smoking habits but were, on the average, of substantially different ages as well. Then it would not be fair to compare their lung cancer incidence as if differences in smoking were all that mattered, since we know that age is also important—the older one gets the higher the likelihood is of developing lung cancer. In order to eliminate this bias we have to determine as a standard of comparison an *expected rate* instead of an actual rate. To do this, we might calculate, for example, what lung cancer incidence rate would be expected in nonsmokers, as before, but now assuming that they were of the same age composition as that of each group of smokers. The method for computing this expected rate involves what is called *age adjustment*, or *age standardization.* This will be discussed further in Chapter 11.

An example of a morbidity ratio comparison using an expected rate is shown in Fig. 2-1. In the Framingham Heart Study men and women in five different blood pressure level groups were compared with one another with respect to the subsequent incidence of coronary heart disease during 8 years. Morbidity ratios were used with an expected rate as a standard of comparison, set at 100 percent. The expected rate was that observed in the whole population, but age-adjusted so that it could be applied fairly to the particular blood pressure group under consideration.

In the figure it can be seen, for example, that for those persons with the lowest systolic blood pressure levels, less than 120 mm Hg, the observed incidence was $^{10}/_{629}$. The expected incidence, based on the experience of the whole population, was $^{30.7}/_{629}$. The ratio of these rates is $^{10}/_{30.7}$, or 33 percent. In contrast to the low incidence in the low blood pressure group, the incidence in the highest group, those with a systolic blood pressure of at least 180 mm Hg, was 223 percent of the expected incidence.

Quantitative Attributes

In considering counts, proportions, and rates we have been dealing with qualitative differences between people—presence or absence of disease, or possession of one versus another attribute. Other characteristics of groups that must be considered lie on a quantitative scale. These characteristics include such measures as height, weight, blood pressure, antibody titer, and diameter of tuberculin skin-test reaction. Epidemiology requires appropriate measures so that groups can be described and compared with respect to these quantitative attributes.

In discussing such measures, one must mention some concepts that are usually presented in books or courses on statistics or biostatistics (see Ipsen and Feigl, 1970). In this introduction to epidemiology it is not necessary to present statistical aspects in great detail, but certain basic measures do deserve mention. Parenthetically, it might be well to remark that one need not be highly

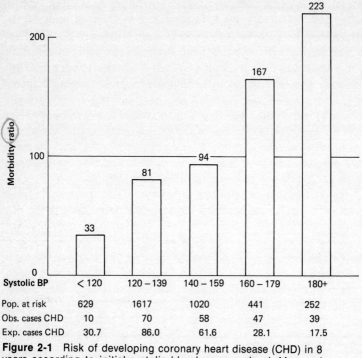

Systolic BP	< 120	120 – 139	140 – 159	160 – 179	180+
Pop. at risk	629	1617	1020	441	252
Obs. cases CHD	10	70	58	47	39
Exp. cases CHD	30.7	86.0	61.6	28.1	17.5

Figure 2-1 Risk of developing coronary heart disease (CHD) in 8 years according to initial systolic blood pressure level. Men and women, ages 30–59 years at entry. Framingham Heart Study. *(Reproduced, by permission, from Kagan et al., 1963.)*

talented in mathematics to understand or carry out epidemiologic studies. While some studies in epidemiology do require sophisticated statistical methods, most problems can be handled well by the simple quantitative measures described here.

Distributions   The most complete summary of a quantitative measurement made on a group of persons is the *distribution.* The distribution tells either how many or what proportion of the group were found to have each value (or each small range of values) out of all the possible values that the quantitative measure can have. In addition, the counts or proportions (or percentages) may be cumulated by adding each successive amount to all those that preceded it.

A distribution of serum uric acid values for 1,734 nonsmoking white men, ages 40–49, is shown in Table 2-1. Note that both numbers and percentages are shown for both the distribution and cumulative distribution.

A distribution may be displayed graphically as a histogram, in which bars represent the numbers or proportions of subjects in each "class interval." The uric acid distribution in Table 2-1 is shown in Fig. 2-2 as a histogram. Note that in plotting a histogram the *area* of each bar communicates the number or proportion of subjects represented. If all bars represent class intervals of the same width, then the area is proportional to the height. If some class intervals or bars are wider, as are the extreme right and left bars in Fig. 2-2, their height must be scaled down proportionally.

Another way to display a distribution is by plotting a series of points. Each point shows the midpoint of an interval and the number or proportion of subjects falling into that interval. The points may be connected by straight lines, yielding a polygon, or they may be

Table 2-1   Distribution and Cumulative Distribution of Serum Uric Acid Concentrations: Nonsmoking Men, Ages 40–49

Serum uric acid (mg/100cc)	Distribution		Cumulative distribution	
	Number	Percent	Number	Percent
1.0–2.9	10	0.6	10	0.6
3.0–3.9	68	3.9	78	4.5
4.0–4.9	315	18.2	393	22.7
5.0–5.9	565	32.6	958	55.3
6.0–6.9	431	24.8	1,389	80.1
7.0–7.9	229	13.2	1,618	93.3
8.0–8.9	85	4.9	1,703	98.2
9.0–11.9	31	1.8	1,734	100.0
Total	1,734	100.0		

Mean = 5.93 mg/100 cc
Standard Deviation = 1.31 mg/100 cc
Range = 1.32 to 11.12, or 9.8 mg/100 cc
Median = 5.84 mg/100 cc
Interquartile Range = 5.07 to 6.79, or 1.72 mg/100 cc
Source: Kaiser-Permanente multiphasic examination data, 1964–1968, tabulated by A. B. Siegelaub, M.S.

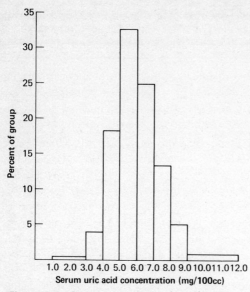

Figure 2-2 Percentage distribution of serum uric acid levels in Table 2-1, displayed as a histogram.

connected so as to form a smooth curve. The uric acid distribution in Table 2-1 is shown as a curve in Fig. 2-3.

Cumulative distributions are usually shown graphically by curves. Fig. 2-4 shows the cumulative distribution curve for the same uric acid data.

Means The *mean*, or arithmetic average, is one of the so-called measures of central tendency of the values for the whole group. It is computed by adding all the individual values together and dividing by the number in the group. When one wishes to compare two or more groups, it may be cumbersome to compare their entire distributions. Comparing means is much simpler. In many cases, for comparative purposes, the mean is a reasonably good representation of the group's values, and it can be expressed with just one number.

It should always be remembered though that the mean is only one feature of a distribution and that two differently shaped distributions may have the same mean. It is often important to know more about the distribution than just the mean. In some cases we may be most interested in knowing how many people are at one extreme of the distribution.

Standard Deviations A good supplement to the mean in describing a group is the *standard deviation*, which is a measure of dispersion or variation. One way to compute it is to (1) square the difference between each value and the mean, (2) add the squared differences, (3) divide that sum by the total number of values minus one, and (4) find the square root of the result of (3). The mean tells where the values for a group are centered. The standard deviation is a summary of how widely dispersed the values are around this center. The standard deviation is also needed in comparing means of different groups to see how likely it is that a difference between two means could have occurred by chance, using statistical significance tests.

Figure 2-3 Percentage distribution of serum uric acid levels in Table 2-1, displayed as a curve.

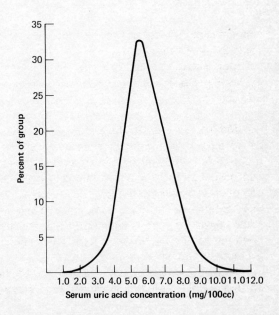

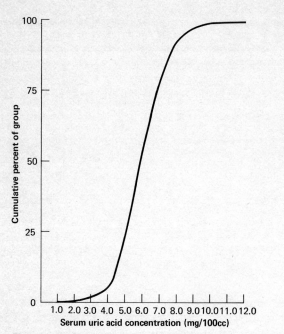

Figure 2-4 Cumulative percentage distribution of serum uric acid levels in Table 2-1, displayed as a curve.

Ranges The *range* of a distribution, the difference between the lowest value and the highest value observed, is, of course, another measure of dispersion. It is often less valuable than the standard deviation, however, since it only tells us about two members of a group. An extremely high or low value may be due to a measurement error.

Quantiles: Values That Divide a Group into Equal Parts Another way to describe a group on a quantitative scale or to classify each member of a group on such a scale is to divide the group into *quantiles*, or equal subgroups, along the scale. The simplest division is into two parts—the lower half and the upper half. The point on the scale that divides the group in this way is called the *median*. In the uric acid distribution shown in Table 2-1 the median value is 5.84 mg/100 cc. (When the median lies within an interval, e.g., between

5.0 and 6.0, we interpolate to estimate just where it lies). One-half of the group has values this high or higher and one-half has values this low or lower. Note that the median value can also be read from the cumulative distribution curve (Fig. 2-4) by seeing what uric acid value corresponds to the 50 percent point on the curve.

Just as one can compare two groups by their means, so one can also compare them by their medians. Medians are less often used than means but they have a few virtues that make them very useful in certain situations. One such situation is when a group has a few members with extreme values. The mean is substantially affected by these extreme values but the median is not. Suppose one wishes to summarize the weights of 22 women attending an obesity clinic. All but one are evenly distributed from 180 to 220 lb (i.e., 180, 182, 184, etc.). One is the fat lady in a traveling circus who weighs 420 lb. When she leaves, the mean weight of the clinic patients will drop by 10 lb, but the median will drop by only 1 lb. Medians are affected little by extreme values.

Another virtue of the median is its usefulness when some values are missing, but known to be above or below a certain level. Suppose one wishes to compare the age at death of two groups of fifty-year-old women exposed to different amounts of ionizing radiation. If one uses the mean age at death, then one must wait until all members of each group die. Conclusions cannot be drawn from the mean age of just some of the deaths, since an early difference between the two groups may be later counterbalanced by a difference in the opposite direction. By the time all the women have died, it is very probable that the investigator will also be dead or no longer interested in the study. Thus it is important to have an earlier answer. The median age at death is one such early measure, since it may be determined when only half the women in each group have died.

Groups may be divided into more than two parts. Three equal parts are known as *terciles*, four equal parts as *quartiles*, five as *quintiles*, ten as *deciles.* The finest division commonly used is into 100 parts, or *percentiles.* Percentiles are often useful for ranking individuals in relation to the total group. (Note that the borderlines between any divisions may be read from the cumulative distribution curve.)

Just as groups can be compared with respect to their medians, they can also be compared as to their borderlines between quartiles, and so on. Similarly, persons in the upper quartile of a value can be compared with those in each of the other quartiles. Also, one may wish to have a measure of dispersion in a group analogous to the standard deviation. The size of the interval between two percentiles, e.g., the 20th and 80th, can be used. One such measure of spread is the *interquartile range*, the interval between the top of the lowest quartile and the bottom of the highest quartile. Note that the interquartile range can easily be read off of a cumulative distribution curve as in Fig. 2-4.

Quantiles may prove very helpful in determining which of two quantitative variables has a stronger relationship to disease. In a particular population group the incidence of coronary heart disease may increase a certain amount with each 20-mm-Hg increase in systolic blood pressure and a different amount with each 20 mg/100 cc increase in serum cholesterol, but this tells us nothing of the relative importance of the two attributes since the units of measurement for blood pressure and cholesterol are completely different, and not at all comparable. A more appropriate contrast would be to note how much the incidence of coronary heart disease increases as one moves up the scale of each measurement by quantile divisions such as deciles or quartiles.

A good example of such a comparison is shown in Fig. 2-5. In the Framingham Heart Study two serum lipid measures, cholesterol and the cholesterol/phospholipid ratio, were compared to determine which was the better predictor of the subsequent development of coronary heart disease. The study population was divided into quartiles of each of the two lipid values. As shown by the morbidity ratios in the figure, the risk of coronary heart disease was clearly related to cholesterol, the incidence being distinctly higher in each successive quartile. In contrast, the increase in risk with increasing quartile of cholesterol/phospholipid ratio was slight, showing that the latter measure was a distinctly inferior predictor.

Epidemiologic Measurements in Perspective

In summary, epidemiology requires that groups of people be described and compared in a quantitative fashion. However, the

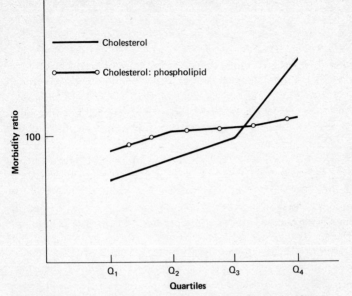

Figure 2-5   Risk of developing coronary heart disease in 10 years in subjects classified into quartiles of cholesterol and cholesterol/phospholipid ratio. Men, ages 30–59 years at entry. Framingham Heart Study. *(Reproduced in modified form, by permission, from Kannel et al., 1964.)*

particular characteristics of interest may be either qualitative or quantitative in nature.

When qualitative attributes are considered, persons with a particular attribute are counted, and the proportion of the total group studied that they constitute is determined. Since disease is the main concern of epidemiology, proportions of groups with disease or rates of disease are given primary attention. Disease rates are usually considered with respect to time. Disease present at one particular time is measured by a prevalence rate. Disease developing over a period of time is measured by an incidence rate.

Comparing disease rates among different groups is of primary importance. These comparisons are often expressed as differences between rates or as ratios of one rate to another.

Quantitative attributes are also important. It is often necessary to consider the entire distribution of the quantitative measure in a group. However, this distribution may be described in a summary fashion by such measures as the mean and standard deviation. Breaking the group into equal parts according to ranking on a quantitative scale (quantiles) serves many useful purposes.

Obviously, the measurements described in this chapter do not exhaust the repertory of the epidemiologist. Other measurements have been used, and new ones will be invented for specific purposes. The simple measures described are established, time-tested, and widely understood.

REFERENCES

Hammond, E. C. Smoking in relation to death rates of one million men and women, *Epidemiological Approaches to the Study of Cancer and Other Chronic Diseases*, edited by W. Haenszel, National Cancer Institute Monograph 19. U.S. Department of Health, Education, and Welfare, Bethesda, January 1966, pp. 127–204.

Ipsen, J., and P. Feigl, *Bancroft's Introduction to Biostatistics*, 2d ed. (New York: Harper and Row, 1970), Chaps. 2, 4, 5 and 11.

Kagan, A., W. B. Kannel, T. R. Dawber, and N. Revotskie. 1963. The coronary profile. *Ann. N.Y. Acad. Sci.*, **97**:883–894.

Kannel, W. B., T. R. Dawber, G. D. Friedman, W. E. Glennon, and P. M. McNamara. 1964. Risk factors in coronary heart disease: An evaluation of several serum lipids as predictors of coronary heart disease: the Framingham study. *Ann. Intern. Med.*, **61**:888–899.

Siegel, M., Indices of community health, in *Preventive Medicine* edited by D. Clark and B. MacMahon. (Boston: Little, Brown, 1967), pp. 67–79.

Chapter 3

Observations Used in Epidemiology

A wide variety of observations and measurements have been used by epidemiologists in their efforts to *describe* and *explain* the occurrence of disease in human populations. There are so many factors that influence human health and disease that almost any aspect of persons and their environments may be fair game for study. Depending upon what is being explored, epidemiologic studies may require the collaboration of scientists from other medical specialties and a variety of other disciplines. Ophthalmology, psychology, physical anthropology, bacteriology, and meteorology are just a few examples.

While we need not consider all varieties of data that may be used, certain types of observations recur frequently enough to deserve discussion. Health-care professionals must have some appreciation of the nature and limitations of these data sources. Not only are they used in scientific study, but they also provide the basis for vital decisions in day-to-day patient care.

Measures of Data Quality: Validity and Reliability

Observations or measurements, whether made by man or machine, involve some degree of error. Errors affect two important aspects of data quality—*validity* and *reliability*.

Validity   Validity, or accuracy, is a measure of how closely the observations correspond to the actual state of affairs. As a clinical illustration, consider a patient with a rapid irregular heartbeat due to atrial fibrillation. Measurement of his heart rate by the radial pulse is considered inaccurate or lacking in validity because some heart beats produce a pulse too weak to be felt at the wrist. Compared to the true heart rate the radial pulse rate is *biased* toward lower values, resulting in what is commonly known as a "pulse deficit."

Reliability   Reliability or reproducibility is a measure of how closely a series of observations of exactly the same thing match one another. If the cholesterol concentration of two portions of the same serum specimen is measured in an automated chemical analyzer, the two results should ideally be exactly the same. To the extent that they are not, the analyzer is said to lack reliability.

Effects of Lack of Validity and Reliability

Observations may be highly reliable but invalid. The cholesterol concentration on duplicate specimens may always agree within 5 mg/100 cc. Yet the readings may consistently be about 30 mg/100 cc too high.

This lack of validity does not necessarily rule out the use of the data. In some instances, knowing a person's absolute level of cholesterol may not be as important as knowing how that person ranks in his group. If all the group's values are 30 mg/100 cc too high, each person in the group will still be properly ranked in relation to the others. However, if one wishes to compare the mean cholesterol for that entire group with the mean of another group, for whom serum cholesterol has been measured accurately, the comparison will be unfair or biased.

Now consider the effects of unreliability. If a group of observations is unreliable, most will also be invalid due to departures from the true values. However, if the unreliability is due to fluctuations that center around the true value, then the average or mean of a large series of observations may be quite a valid measure of the true average or mean. In this case many individuals will be improperly ranked relative to one another, if the ranking is based on one measurement for each. However, a comparison of the mean cholesterol of one large group with that of another may be quite fair and unbiased.

Usual Sources of Variation in Measurements

Not all the fluctuations in measurements or observations are attributable to lack of validity or reliability. The attributes themselves usually vary in a variety of ways.

Consider the distribution of blood pressures found in a community survey in which each subject has two measurements made. The major components of variation in the distribution are as follows:

Differences among subgroups—e.g., blacks have higher blood pressures, on the average, than whites; older persons have higher blood pressures than younger ones.

Differences among individuals within a subgroup—e.g., among black men, age 50, some individuals have higher blood pressures than others.

Differences within each individual—due to a variety of influences, each individual's blood pressure varies from one moment to the next. Some of these intraindividual differences may follow a regular pattern, e.g., diurnal variation.

Measurement errors—even if all blood pressures measured were exactly the same, they would appear to vary because of the failings of the observer, be it human or a mechanical device.

Sampling Variation

Another source of error or variation in data, known as *sampling variation*, is due to chance. It can be overcome by studying groups that are sufficiently large.

When we study the occurrence of a disease in a group of men, aged 50–59, in a community, we would like to think that our findings are applicable to all men of that age decade in that community. The findings would undoubtedly be true of all 50-to-59-year-old men in the community if we studied all of them, but we usually have to take a sample. If the sample is selected in such a way that all men have an equal chance of being chosen, then we have what is called a *random sample*.

Experience and the laws of probability tell us that the larger the sample that is studied, the more likely are the findings to be representative of the total population. Conversely, the smaller the sample, the more likely we are to be misled. If repeated samples are drawn from a population, the findings in each sample will differ from one another—thus the term, "sampling variation." The larger the sample size, the less the variation, and the less chance of error.

This fact may be readily seen in the classic example of a large bag full of an equal mixture of black and white marbles. If an observer tries to determine what proportion of the marbles are white by pulling out only two marbles, he has a 25 percent probability of picking out two white marbles and concluding erroneously that all the marbles are white. If he pulls out four marbles instead, his chances of getting all white marbles are much less, only 1 in 16, or about 6 percent. One may apply the laws of probability to compute the likelihood of this false conclusion with any size sample; the result corresponds with our intuitive feeling that the more marbles one looks at, the less the chance of concluding that those in the bag are all white.

Thus, the larger the sample or group studied, the less the probability that chance error may occur. Statistical significance tests (such as "t" or chi square tests, and a variety of others described in statistics texts) are used to measure the probability of chance errors, given the size and characteristics of the study population and the question that is being asked. The result of a test of statistical significance is a probability level or "p" value, as frequently seen in medical journal articles. The expression "$p < 0.05$" means that there is less than a 5 percent probability that the observed result could have occurred by chance error.

Clinical Observations

Clinical observations are the primary basis for decisions as to the presence or absence of a particular disease. The most basic clinical observations constitute the clinical history and physical examination. These are usually obtained by physicians, nurses, and other specially trained physicians' assistants.

The means for obtaining a history and physical examination need not be described here, but some comment about their limitations is in order. Many physicians have had memorable experiences in the unreliability of the medical history interview when they were medical students. Consider this all-too-familiar example. In preparation for rounds with the professor of cardiology the student devotes 10 minutes to careful questioning of the patient concerning nocturnal dyspnea and convinces himself that the patient indeed becomes short of breath at night and must sit up in bed in order to breathe more easily. After presenting the history during rounds the next day, the embarrassed student hears the patient tell the professor that he has never been short of breath at night.

The physical examination is no more reliable. If the patient is examined by half a dozen physicians, there will often be one or two who will hear (or not hear) a faint diastolic murmur not heard (or heard) by the others. The same degree of disagreement may be expected concerning the palpability of an elusive spleen. Differences in observer skill cannot be denied. Yet the murmur-hearers and spleen-feelers hold the psychological advantage, and objectivity probably suffers as a result.

Blood pressure, measured with a sphygmomanometer, has been a convenient measurement for the study of observer error in clinical medicine. It is a very sobering experience to be among a group viewing a movie prepared by Wilcox (1961), which shows a series of 14 views of a descending column of mercury in a sphygmomanometer accompanied by Korotkov's sounds amplified from a stethoscope. The group is asked to record the systolic and diastolic pressure for each measurement displayed. Even though all observers are seeing the same column of mercury and hearing the same sounds, the differences in the recorded results are striking. The greatest surprise comes when the viewers, learning that some of the early and late scenes are exactly the same, find discrepancies in their own readings for duplicate measurements.

When the results of a series of blood pressure measurements are tabulated, one human source of error that usually comes to light is *digit preference.* Physicians may tend to record values rounded off to a last digit of 5 or 0, or a preference for even over odd numbers becomes apparent (Fig. 3-1). Also noted has been a tendency to slant borderline values downward to avoid making unpleasant diagnoses.

Observations of Medical Specialists

Physicians in certain medical specialties make particular observations that are supposed to provide highly objective evidence as to the presence or absence of disease. Radiologists have the x-ray, cardiologists have the electrocardiogram, and pathologists have their stained microscopic sections. Implicit in giving a pathologist the last word in a clinicopathologic conference is perhaps the feeling that his observations will not only shed additional light on difficult problems, but that they are more reliable and valid than those of a bedside clinician.

A few of these specialists have made important contributions to our knowledge of the extent of observer variation in medicine. They

Figure 3-1 Percentage distribution of terminal digits on both systolic and diastolic blood pressure readings by an examining physician in the Los Angeles Heart Study. *(Reproduced, by permission, from Chapman, Clark, and Coulson, 1966.)*

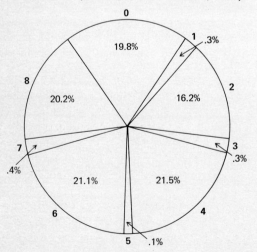

have had the interest and courage to participate in studies to compare observations of the same visual object by different members of the same specialty or to compare duplicate observations by the same individual. The lack of reliability, even in these so-called objective measurements, has been striking.

Perhaps the classic series of studies in this area was carried out by Yerushalmy (1969) and his associates in the field of radiology. In one such study 14,541 entering college students received 70-mm chest photofluorograms. Each film was interpreted twice by two physicians and once by six others. Follow-up study of students with films read as "positive" by more than one reader, was accomplished by 14- by 17-in. chest film interpreted by a group of radiologists. The final interpretation regarding the presence of pulmonary tuberculosis was that 177 students had films that were "roentgenologically positive," 61 were "roentgenologically urgent," and 13 were "clinically active." Each of these cases, of course, had initial films that had been read by eight different readers. The percentages of original readings that were falsely read as negative were as follows:

	False negatives
Roentgenologically positive	26.9%
Roentgenologically urgent	25.4%
Clinically active	25.0%

Thus about one-quarter of all these nontrivial cases were missed the first time by competent x-ray readers.

Another series of 1,256 14- by 17-in. films were interpreted by a group of five competent radiologists and tuberculosis specialists. The number of films read as positive for tuberculosis by each reader was 56, 59, 62, 70, and 109, respectively. "Moreover, the radiologist who selected 109 did not include all those selected by the one who selected only 56." Similarly each reader read a different number as being positive when he read the films a second time. In each case some of the films read as positive once were read as negative by the same reader on another occasion.

The presence or absence of significant disease was not the only subject of inter- and intraobserver disagreement. Commonly accepted descriptive terms for pulmonary lesions such as "active," "inactive," "fibrotic," "soft," "hard," and "cavity" showed great differences among readers. After 2 years of work in trying to develop a reliable classification scheme to describe pulmonary lesions, the group of radiologists concluded that they had failed. "It was disappointing to find that many conferences and much practice, together and apart failed to increase reliability and agreement to a useful degree."

Interpretation of serial roentgenograms, the basis for many clinical decisions about tuberculosis patients, was also found to be grossly inconsistent. In making a judgment as to whether two x-ray films taken at different times showed progression, regression, or stability of disease, two readers disagreed with each other in about one-third of cases and a single reader disagreed with himself in about one-fifth of cases.

Clinical Diagnoses

Diagnoses are inferences or conclusions based on clinical and laboratory observations. Not only may these observations be incorrect, but the reasoning leading to the conclusions may also be in error. Yet even if the observations are complete and accurate and the reasoning is sound, differently trained physicians use different criteria for making the same diagnosis. Also leading to observer variations is the fact that one physician may have access to more laboratory tests or other specialized data. Furthermore, different terms may be used to refer to the same clinical condition, and a single term (e.g., "arteriosclerotic heart disease") may have different meanings to different physicians.

Thus, clinical diagnoses by themselves are indeed undependable indicators of disease for scientific study. Whenever possible, specific criteria should be established for making diagnoses. These criteria should be adhered to carefully and described clearly so that the work may be repeated or evaluated by others.

Medical Chart Review

Both epidemiologic studies and patient care frequently rely upon the review and abstracting of information from medical records. Just as is found for other types of observations, the reading of charts involves substantial amounts of error. Even if the information is relatively complete and the various handwritings are legible, two chart readers will extract differing information. Usually, however, matters are much worse, with missing information and cryptic or illegible physicians' notes.

Disease Reporting

Physicians are legally required to report certain diseases to the local public health authorities at the time of diagnosis. The primary purpose of this is to detect the onset of epidemics of certain serious diseases and to provide information so that appropriate community-wide control measures can be undertaken. In addition to their usefulness in disease control these data may also be used to measure disease incidence in the community.

Despite official requirements, many diseases are underreported. For example it has been estimated that, despite the mounting concern over the recent epidemic of venereal disease, only one-fourth of all cases are reported. Desire to avoid social stigma for patients, the pressures of other work, and laxity are among the reasons that have been given for underreporting.

This is not only the case with regard to certain infectious diseases. In the 1950's and 1960's two large agencies, the American Medical Association and the U.S. Food and Drug Administration carried out special programs to encourage physicians to report instances of suspected adverse drug reactions. The purposes of these programs were to obtain some measure of the frequency of occurrence of various drug reactions and to provide a means of receiving early warnings of as yet unsuspected side effects of drugs. The response of physicians was quite disappointing. By and large, busy physicians do not wish to take the time to fill out the reporting forms. In a study of various approaches to detecting adverse drug reactions in a hospital, Cluff et al. (1964) judged a system whereby physicians were to fill out a drug reaction card at the time of discharge to be "completely unsatisfactory," since intensive daily surveillance of just one service yielded four times as many reactions as were listed by report card from the entire hospital.

Death Certificates and Mortality Statistics

Mortality data for nations, states, and communities, as obtained from death certificates, have played an important role in epidemiologic research for more than a century. Many major problems and inaccuracies are associated with death certificates. (See Feinstein, 1968, for detailed discussion.) Nevertheless, they constitute a widely implemented collection of data about fatal illnesses that can be used to study disease occurrence on a local, national, or international scale.

     Death certificate diagnoses are usually clinical diagnoses and are thus subject to all the vagaries described above. In addition, the patient may have had several diseases contributing to his death, but under current procedures, only one underlying cause is to be selected. Before 1949 in the United States, coding rules automatically led to the choice of one underlying cause out of several possibilities. For example, if both diabetes mellitus and heart disease were listed on the death certificate, diabetes was coded as the underlying cause even if the doctor felt that heart disease was more to blame. Starting in 1949, the physician was asked to indicate the underlying cause. While this may have been an improvement, it resulted in some sudden changes in apparent mortality rates (e.g., a drop in diabetes mortality, as would be expected); it also forced physicians to oversimplify many complex situations where multiple causes might have been involved. For this reason, many authorities have urged the adoption of a multiple-cause coding system for death certificates. If mortality statistics are to become more meaningful, it would be helpful if physicians were trained in uniform and proper procedures for filling out death certificates.

     Other changes in diagnostic classifications have been made in the *International Classification of Diseases*, now in its eighth revision, leading to abrupt changes in reported mortality rates for the diseases affected. Studies of time trends in disease mortality must take into account these coding changes as well as the technological advances that lead to increased diagnoses of particular conditions and changes in the fashion of allocating deaths to one disease instead of another. Fig. 3-2, from a study by Reid and Evans (1970), shows time trends in mortality rates for nephritis, hypertension, and

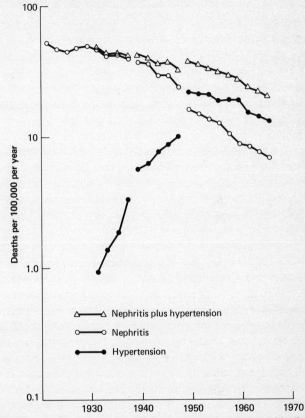

Figure 3-2 Mortality rates from nephritis, hypertension, and both combined, among males aged 45–54 years in England and Wales, from 1931–1966. *(Reproduced, by permission, from Reid and Evans, 1970.)*

both combined, among men ages 45–54 in England and Wales, and illustrates several of these factors. The gaps in the curves reflect changes in disease classification. The sharp rise in the death rate for hypertension between 1931 and 1950 probably reflects the increased use of the sphygmomanometer and an increased awareness of the importance of hypertension. The reciprocal changes in hypertension and nephritis deaths may represent an increasing tendency to attribute uremia to kidney damage produced by hypertension rather than by inflammation.

Responses to Questionnaires

The clinical history is only one of many kinds of data that may be obtained by questionnaires. Data relating to social status or exposures to environmental hazards can also be obtained in this manner.

It does not seem necessary to belabor the frailties of human observations and their written or oral communications any further, except to encourage again a reasonably skeptical attitude toward the results of questionnaire studies and to show some examples of problems commonly encountered.

Nonresponse If given a choice, a substantial proportion of individuals will not answer questions. In 1971 a questionnaire was mailed to 8,250 Kaiser Foundation Health Plan members participating in a study to evaluate periodic checkups involving multiphasic screening. Because of the incomplete response to one mailing, four subsequent mailings were sent out to nonrespondents. The percentage of the total group responding to each mailing is shown in Table 3-1. The final nonresponse rate of 20.4 percent (100 percent minus 79.6 percent) is not at all unusual for a mailed questionnaire.

Nonresponse can also occur under more controlled or supervised conditions. As part of a multiphasic examination at Kaiser-Permanente, patients are given a self-administered questionnaire containing a series of questions about their smoking habits. The answers to the questions about smoking were used to classify examinees in a study of the characteristics of smokers and nonsmokers (Friedman et al., 1972). In doing so it was found that about 12.7 percent of 111,024 persons did not answer at least one of the crucial questions about present or past smoking habits.

Nonresponse would not constitute a serious problem if it merely reduced the number of subjects available for study; however, it may also lead to a biased study sample if the respondents and nonrespondents differ with respect to health or some other characteristic being studied. Unfortunately, this is frequently the case.

Table 3-1   Response to Five Mailings of a Questionnaire by 8,250 Kaiser Health Plan Members*

Mailing	Percentage of total study group responding
First	43.4
Second	15.4
Third	8.6
Fourth	7.0
Fifth	5.2
Total	79.6

*Data tabulated by Barbara A. Campbell, M.A.

Inconsistent or Otherwise Unusable Responses   It is surprising how often persons will answer both "yes" and "no" to the same questionnaire item or provide otherwise inconsistent responses. In the study of smoking just referred to 2.3 percent of subjects did not indicate that they smoked cigarettes, but then gave a positive response to some duration of smoking or quantity of cigarettes smoked. Because of this and other serious inconsistencies, plus the omissions described above, 16.5 percent, or about one-sixth of the total subjects, had to be eliminated.

Overreporting of Disease Symptoms   Patients who either deny or exaggerate disease symptoms are well known to physicians. In a study of the reliability of a self-administered questionnaire (Collen et al., 1969) it was found that on the average, one-fifth of persons who answered "yes" to a symptom question the first time, denied the symptom when the questionnaire was administered again at the same examination. Physicians who perform follow-up examinations after patients have answered a symptom questionnaire often find that positive responses to questions about serious symptoms either cannot be substantiated or appear nonsignificant upon careful history-taking. As an example of the likely overreporting of symptoms on a self-administered questionnaire, 15.9 percent of

1,950 girls, ages 15–19, taking Kaiser-Permanente multiphasic examinations, answered "yes" to the following question describing symptoms almost pathognomonic of angina pectoris: "In the past year have you had repeated pain (or pressure or tight feeling) in your chest when you walked fast or uphill and that left after a few minutes rest?"

Presenting Oneself in a Favorable Light   This is such a universal trait that it hardly needs to be mentioned except that it can introduce systematic biases into epidemiologic studies. Persons tend to deny venereal disease and drug abuse and underestimate their alcohol consumption.

Household Surveys

Information about medical conditions and other pertinent social and personal characteristics is frequently obtained by household interview survey. Assessments of health and social problems by survey may be the basis of determining priorities for community or national policy. Thus, the limitations of this study method should be well understood.

Problems associated with survey data and the techniques of obtaining representative samples of individuals for questioning have been a major concern of social scientists. In the health field, the *National Health Survey* (NHS) has been authorized by the United States Congress to carry out surveys by the household interview method since 1957. In the course of this work NHS scientists have carried out important methodologic studies to determine the accuracy of interview-acquired information.

In one such study (Madow, 1967), patients' reporting of chronic conditions was compared to the chronic conditions recorded by physicians in their medical records during a 1-year period. Overall, 45.3 percent or almost half the chronic conditions recorded by the physicians were not reported by the patients despite the fact that patients were given a fairly comprehensive checklist of conditions to jog their memories.

Thus, interview data about illness are apt to be incomplete. As might be expected, conditions for which the patient made more frequent doctor visits were more apt to be reported, as were those for which a doctor was seen more recently. Furthermore, conditions were more likely to be reported in an interview if they affected the person's way of life, for example, by causing pain or worry or limitations in his work or in what he could eat or drink.

Laboratory Data

Mechanical, electrical, and chemical measurements are also subject to error. Well-run clinical laboratories maintain continuing quality control programs to monitor the validity and reliability of their measurements. When significant errors occur, monitoring permits institution of prompt corrective action.

Yet, even with the most careful quality control, significant errors occur, due both to known and unknown factors. Many of these factors cannot be controlled within the laboratory. Only in the past decade, for example, did it become generally known that exposure of a blood specimen to light would cause a breakdown of bilirubin and significantly lower the serum bilirubin concentration measured in the laboratory. Similarly, ingestion of a variety of drugs can affect the measurement of important blood constituents. A well-known example is the effect of iodide-containing drugs on the protein-bound iodine test of thyroid function.

STUDYING RELATIONSHIPS IN IMPERFECT DATA: THE VALUE OF INVESTIGATING LARGE GROUPS

This section is, to the author, one of the most important in this book. It will attempt to bridge a serious gap in understanding and communication between the scientifically minded clinician and the epidemiologist.

As will be developed more fully in the next chapter, one of the primary concerns of the epidemiologist, like other scientists, is the study of *relationships.* The epidemiologist focuses on relationships between diseases and other human or environmental attributes by studying population groups.

The clinician focuses on the individual patient and strives to obtain complete and accurate information, in order to provide the best possible diagnosis and treatment. In his appropriate concern for the patient's welfare, he can tolerate few avoidable errors in this information. Accustomed to high standards in his pursuit of information and the expenditure, if necessary, of hundreds of dollars per patient in laboratory tests and specialized diagnostic procedures, he becomes intolerant of the use of relatively low-quality data such as questionnaires or death certificates in epidemiologic studies.

A case in point is the difficulty in convincing some neurologists of the validity of epidemiologic studies of stroke that do not include an evaluation of all study subjects by a neurologist. Neurologists spend years learning the subtleties of the neurological examination and the fine points of differentiating strokes from a variety of other neurological conditions (many of which are quite rare). To many physicians with such a background it is inconceivable that one would undertake a scientific study of stroke based, say, on identification of cases simply by asking, "Have you ever had a stroke?"

Yet in a study of a large population, the human and financial resources to provide a neurologist's examination for all subjects are not available now, nor will they be in the foreseeable future. So let's compromise and have any ill persons in whom the attending physician suspects a stroke evaluated by a neurologist. This approach is more workable and can be employed in special intensive population studies such as the Framingham Study (described in Chap. 8). Yet even there, practical difficulties arise; if a person has a stroke which is rapidly fatal or which occurs out of town, he will probably not be seen by a neurologist.

The epidemiologist is not in favor of bad data. He wants the best he can get. But experience has shown that he can discern important relationships, even in data of relatively poor quality because studying large groups provides power to overcome error. With some validity to the data and large enough numbers of study subjects to minimize sampling error, one may still derive some valuable information from poor quality data.

Consider the following numerical example. Suppose that we wish to determine whether there is a relationship of stroke to hypertension and we can only use a questionnaire which asks, "Have you ever had a stroke?" and "Have you ever had high blood pressure?" The questionnaire is administered to 10,000 persons, ages 65–74. Let us postulate that the true state of affairs for this population happens to be that 200 persons have had a stroke and 2,000 have had high blood pressure. Of the stroke cases, 150 had high blood pressure. The *true* population breakdown is shown in Table 3-2.

A slight digression here may be of value to the reader who is unfamiliar with the presentation of data in a "two-by-two" or "fourfold" table, frequently used in epidemiology and exemplified by Table 3-2. These tables show the relationship of one "yes-or-no," or dichotomous, variable to another. The presence or absence of one disease or characteristic is indicated at the left and the presence or absence of the other is shown at the top.

Table 3-2 shows how the population is divided in the four possible ways according to each of the two characteristics. The number, 150, in the upper left corner indicates that there are 150 persons with both a history of stroke and of hypertension. The number, 1,850, to the right of the 150, represents 1,850 persons with a history of hypertension but no history of stroke. The sum of 150 and 1,850, or 2,000, is shown at the far upper right and represents all persons with a history of hypertension. The 8,000 persons without a history of hypertension are shown in the second row. Fifty of the 8,000, on the left, have a history of stroke. The 7,950, next to them, do not have a history of stroke. The total of 50 plus 7,950, or 8,000, is shown to the right. Totals of the columns are shown below and represent the 200 persons with a history of stroke and the 9,800

Table 3-2 "True" Breakdown of a Population of 10,000 Persons, Ages 65–74, According to the Presence or Absence of a History of Hypertension and a History of Stroke (Fictitious Data)

| | | Stroke history (True) | | |
		Present	Absent	Total
Hypertension history	Present	150	1,850	2,000
(True)	Absent	50	7,950	8,000
	Total	200	9,800	10,000

without. The grand total of the population, or 10,000, is shown at the lower right-hand corner.

Returning now to the argument at hand, the prevalence of a history of stroke in those with a history of high blood pressure is $150/_{2,000}$ or 7.5 percent. The prevalence of a stroke history in those without a hypertension history is $50/_{8,000}$ or 0.625 percent. Thus, if one could only know the true situation, one would find that those with high blood pressure in the past had $7.5/_{0.625}$, or 12 times, the likelihood of the nonhypertensives, of having a history of stroke.

Now let us estimate that our questionnaire only elicits positive responses to the stroke question from 160, or four-fifths, of the stroke cases and, in addition, 196, or 2 percent, of the 9,800 nonstroke cases answered "yes" to the stroke question by mistake. Let us also assume that only one-half of hypertensives were aware of, and reported, their elevated blood pressure and that 5 percent of nonhypertensives erroneously reported that they were hypertensive.

As a result of these errors, some of the persons from each "true" category will be moved to each of the four "reported" categories. For example, consider the 150 persons with *true* strokes and *true* hypertension. Only half report their hypertension. Of the 75 reporting either hypertension or nonhypertension one-fifth do not report their stroke. So the 150 "true" stroke cases with hypertension will be distributed into the four "reported" categories as shown in Table 3-3.

Table 3-3   Parceling Out the 150 Persons with a "True" History of Both Stroke and Hypertension into Four Categories According to What They Will Report on the Questionnaire (Fictitious data)

| | | Stroke history (reported) | |
		Present	Absent
Hypertension history (reported)	Present	60	15
	Absent	60	15

One may go through this exercise with each of the other three "true" categories and divide each into the four "reported" categories. If one then adds all the persons in each of the "reported" categories, the (rounded) result is as shown in Table 3-4.

Now the observed prevalence of a history of stroke in prior hypertensives is $^{88}/_{1,400}$, or 6.3 percent. This is about twice the 3.1 percent prevalence ($^{268}/_{8,600}$) in prior normotensives. *Despite the poor quality of the data, the relationship between hypertension and stroke, while not as strong as in reality, may still be perceived.* Thus, the study of relationships in groups of people can, to some degree, overcome certain kinds of error.

This is not an argument for using poor data when better are obtainable. One must always be aware of the limitations of his data and how inaccuracies and biases may affect his results. In the example it was assumed that the failure to report hypertension was equally true of persons with and without stroke. If stroke affected memory so as to further diminish the reporting of hypertension in the stroke case group, then the study might have missed the stroke-hypertension relationship completely, or might even have led to the opposite conclusion. Thus, data can be, and often are so bad as to be unrevealing or even misleading, despite large numbers.

The example given illustrates another epidemiologic principle. Where relationships are observed in data with an appreciable number of misclassified subjects (e.g., persons with a disease classified as not having it), the results are conservative. That is, the

Table 3-4 Findings in the Total Population Based upon What They Report on the Questionnaire (Fictitious Data)

		Stroke history (reported)		
		Present	Absent	Total
Hypertension history (reported)	Present	88	1,312	1,400
	Absent	268	8,332	8,600
	Total	356	9,644	10,000

relationship in real life is greater than is revealed by the data. In the above example the misclassifications of patients regarding their blood pressure or stroke status reduced an actual twelvefold increase of stroke in hypertensives to an observed twofold increase.

Nevertheless, the study of large groups allows one to detect important relationships, using poor data that are intolerable in conscientious patient care. This, then, is the explanation to the clinician of the seeming tolerance of epidemiology for inadequate data.

REFERENCES

Chapman, J. M., V. A. Clark, and A. H. Coulson. 1966. Problems of measurement in blood pressure surveys: Inter-observer differences in blood pressure determinations. *Am. J. Epidemiology*, **84**:483–494.

Cluff, L. E., G. F. Thornton, and L. G. Seidl. 1964. Studies on the epidemiology of adverse drug reactions: I. Methods of surveillance. *J. Am. Med. Assoc.*, **188**:976–983.

Collen, M. F., J. L. Cutler, A. B. Siegelaub, R. L. Cella. 1969. Reliability of a self-administered questionnaire. *Arch. Intern. Med.*, **123**:664–681.

Feinstein, A. R. 1968. Clinical epidemiology. II. The identification rates of disease. *Ann. Intern. Med.*, **69**:1037–1061.

Friedman, G. D., C. C. Seltzer, A. B. Siegelaub, R. Feldman, and M. F. Collen. 1972. Smoking among white, black and yellow men and women: Kaiser-Permanente Multiphasic Health examination data, 1964–1968. *Am. J. Epidemiology*, **96**:23–35.

Madow, W. G., Interview data on chronic conditions compared with information derived from medical records. National Center for Health Statistics Report, Ser. 2, No. 23, U.S. Department of Health, Education, and Welfare, 1967.

Reid, D. D., and J. G. Evans. 1970. New drugs and changing mortality from non-infectious disease in England and Wales. *Brit. Med. Bull.*, **26**:191–196.

Wilcox, J. 1961. Observer factors in the measurement of blood pressure. *Nursing Research*, **10**:4–20.

Yerushalmy, J. 1969. The statistical assessment of the variability in observer perception and description of roentgenographic pulmonary shadows. *Radiol. Clin. N. Amer.*, **7**:381–392.

Chapter 4

Basic Methods of Study

In the two preceding chapters the reader has been introduced to the data employed in epidemiology and the basic measurements that are used to describe groups of persons. It is now appropriate to consider the major types of epidemiological investigation. Each type of study uses these tools in a particular way and has a unique logical framework. In addition, each type of study is especially appropriate for the unique circumstances surrounding any particular investigation—the aims of the investigation, the populations available for study, and the human and financial resources that can be brought to bear on the problem.

Relationships

Much of the effort of medical scientists in understanding the etiology of disease and developing appropriate therapies involves a study of the relationship of one type of event or characteristic or "variable" to another. Consider the following questions as examples:

Does exposure to cold wet weather predispose to the common cold?
What is the influence of the serum potassium concentration on the contractility of the heart?
Is obesity related to the occurrence of gallstones?
What is the effect of vitamin C deprivation on wound healing?
Which part of the hemoglobin molecule carries the oxygen?
Does BCG vaccination provide protection against pulmonary tuberculosis?

In Table 4-1 these questions are listed together with the relationship that should be studied to help answer each. In a two-variable relationship one is usually considered the *independent* variable, which affects the other, or *dependent*, variable.

The relationships that are studied need not be only between one variable and a second. Often, the investigator must be concerned with the interrelationship of three or more variables. For example, in order to better understand the relationship of potassium to the force of cardiac contraction, calcium concentration must also be taken into account. Whether or not obesity is related to gallstone occurrence may depend on racial characteristics and the type of diet eaten, both of which must be considered and assessed as additional independent variables.

Observational versus Experimental Studies

There are two basic approaches to investigating the relationship between variables. In *observational* studies, nature is allowed to take its course and changes or differences in one characteristic are related to changes or differences in the other, if any. In *experimental* studies, the investigator actually intervenes and makes one variable change and then sees what happens to the other. In doing so he tries, as much as possible, not to allow other important variables to affect the outcome. By controlling the experimental situation, he may conclude that the intervention or manipulation of the in-

Table 4-1 Examples of Relationships Studied in Order to Answer Certain Questions

Question	Suggests study of the relationship between variables	
	Independent variables	Dependent variables
Does exposure to cold wet weather predispose to the common cold?	Daily weather conditions	Incidence of common cold
What is the influence of the serum potassium concentration on the contractility of the heart?	Serum potassium concentration	Stroke output of the heart
Is obesity related to the occurrence of gallstones?	Skinfold thickness	Prevalence of gallstones
What is the effect of vitamin C deprivation on wound healing?	Vitamin C content of the diet	Tensile strength of healing wounds
Which part of the hemoglobin molecule carries the oxygen?	Portion of hemoglobin molecule	Affinity for oxygen
Does BCG vaccination provide protection against pulmonary tuberculosis?	Presence or absence of vaccination	Incidence of tuberculosis

dependent variable actually affected, or caused the change in, the dependent variable.

Epidemiology includes both observational and experimental studies. An example of an epidemiologic experiment was the large-scale field trial of poliomyelitis vaccine in which two large groups of children, comparable in all important respects (e.g., age, health, socioeconomic status, and likelihood of exposure to poliomyelitis virus) received vaccine and placebo, respectively, with follow-up to measure the subsequent incidence of poliomyelitis (described in Chap. 9).

Because of the difficulties of performing well-controlled experiments on human populations and the availability of an abundance of observational data, epidemiologists have tended to concentrate on observational studies. In doing so they have tried to "control" the important extraneous variables by their data-analysis methods. Also, they are always on the lookout for "natural experiments"— spontaneous occurrences which approximate experiments by virtue of a change in only one independent variable that is apparently unaccompanied by changes in other important variables. An example might be the sudden graded exposure to ionizing radiation received in 1945 by the population of Hiroshima, which has permitted the study of the relationship of different doses of radiation exposure to the subsequent development of a variety of diseases.

Such natural experiments are rare (thank goodness) and the observational epidemiologist has to rely on other techniques and criteria for determining the possible effects of additional variables.

Observational studies fall into two main categories, descriptive and analytic. These studies, in turn, may be subdivided into cross-sectional or prevalence studies, case-control studies, and incidence or cohort studies, depending on the groups of persons investigated and the time relationships involved. (Case-control studies are probably best included only in the analytic category.) These will be described subsequently. Attention will also be paid to defining and clarifying the relationship between prospective and retrospective studies due to the confusion that revolves around this distinction.

Descriptive versus Analytic Studies

There are two fundamental objectives of observational epidemiologic studies. One is to *describe* the occurrence of disease or disease-related phenomena in populations. The other is to *explain* the observed pattern of occurrence of disease. Seeking the latter objective involves the identification of causal or etiological factors.

Descriptive studies usually involve the determination of the incidence, prevalence, and mortality rates for diseases in large population groups, according to basic group characteristics such as age, sex, race, and geographic area. In this way, the general distribution of disease in the population is described.

Studies attempting to explain disease are often referred to as *analytic* studies. The starting point for an analytic study is often a descriptive finding that raises certain questions or suggests certain hypotheses that require further investigation. With analytic studies the investigator has a specific question or group of questions in mind that he sets about to answer.

The distinction between descriptive and analytic studies is not clear-cut. A large-scale descriptive study may (perhaps unexpectedly) provide abundant and impressive data that give a clear answer to a specific question. In an analytic study, designed to answer specific questions, data collected incidentally may be of great descriptive interest and raise further questions for investigation.

Despite this fuzziness, it is often useful to categorize epidemiologic studies in this manner. Descriptive studies usually involve a more diffuse, superficial, or general view of a disease problem. Analytic studies narrow down on a specific question and may require a more rigorous study design and data analysis.

Prevalence or Cross-Sectional Studies

Prevalence, or *cross-sectional*, studies examine the relationships between diseases and other characteristics or variables of interest as they exist in a defined population at one particular time. The presence or absence of disease and the presence or absence of the other variables (or, if they are quantitative, their level) are determined in each member of the study population or in a representative sample at one particular time. The relationship between a variable and the disease can be examined in two ways, either (1) in terms of the prevalence of disease in different population subgroups defined according to the presence or absence (or level) of the variables or, conversely, (2) in terms of the presence or absence (or level) of the variables in the diseased versus the nondiseased.

Case-Control Studies

Case-control studies are similar to prevalence studies in that they assess the relationship of *existing* disease to other variables or attributes. After the initial identification of cases, that is, location of persons with the disease of interest, a suitable control group or comparison group of persons without the disease is identified. The relationship of an attribute to the disease is examined by comparing the diseased and nondiseased with regard to how frequently the attribute is present or, if quantitative, what the levels of the attribute are in the two groups.

Incidence or Cohort Studies

Instead of measuring the relationship of attributes to existing disease, as do prevalence and case-control studies, *incidence*, or *cohort*, studies look more directly at attributes or factors related to the *development* of disease. A study population free of the disease under investigation is identified at a particular time. The attributes of interest are measured initially in this group of persons, known as a *cohort*. Then, these persons are followed up over a period of time for the development of the disease being studied. The relationship of an attribute to the disease is examined by dividing the population into subgroups according to the presence or absence (or level) of the attribute initially and comparing the subsequent incidence of disease in each of the subgroups.

An Illustrative Example

Prevalence, case-control, and incidence studies are discussed in detail in Chapters 6, 7, and 8, respectively. At this point an example may help to clarify the distinction among these study plans. Suppose we wish to learn whether obesity predisposes to degenerative arthritis of the knees. In a prevalence study we would x-ray the knees of a defined population, perhaps all the adults in a community, and determine degree of obesity by measuring height and weight or skinfold thickness. We would then compare the prevalence of osteoarthritis in population subgroups showing various degrees of obesity. Or, we may wish to contrast the mean skinfold thickness or other obesity measure in those with osteoarthritis and those without.

In a case-control study of this question, we might collect a group of persons with osteoarthritis of the knees hospitalized at a local hospital during the past year. For a control group, we might select for each osteoarthritis case, a person of the same sex and similar age, admitted to the same hospital during the same week for minor elective surgery such as herniorrhaphy or hemorrhoidectomy. We would then compare the recorded heights and weights of the case group with those of the control group to see if, indeed, the osteoarthritis cases were more obese.

To approach this problem by an incidence study, we would go back to a defined adult population and x-ray their knees to exclude persons with existing osteoarthritis. We would then measure skin-fold thickness or height and weight in order to divide the population without osteoarthritis into the obese and nonobese or, preferably, some finer gradations of fatness. We would call them back 10 years later for repeat knee x-rays, which would demonstrate new cases of osteoarthritis. Then we would compare the incidence of osteoarthritis in the various fatness groups.

Remembering our original question, "Does obesity *predispose* to osteoarthritis?" the incidence study approach seems to provide the most direct answer, since we looked for obesity *before* the osteoarthritis developed. The prevalence and case-control studies provided only indirect evidence, since they looked at obesity at the same time as disease. However, the time sequence can often be taken into account in the prevalence and case-control studies. In addition to measuring current weight in persons with and without osteoarthritis we could also have inquired about their weight 10 years ago, or at age 25, or before their knees started to hurt, thus investigating their weight prior to the development of osteoarthritis. The information obtained may not be as accurate as that derived from weighing the subjects initially in an incidence study, but time sequence can be considered in prevalence or case-control studies.

Prospective and Retrospective Studies

The question of time sequence leads naturally into a consideration of the much-discussed *prospective* and *retrospective* studies. It is almost a matter of faith that investigations are unsatisfactory if they are retrospective. One often hears such comments as, "Of course, this study was retrospective, so we can not be confident of the findings."

Before discussing the merits of prospective versus retrospective studies, it is important to clarify their meaning. Actually, much confusion has resulted because the terms are used in two different ways leading to such semantic horrors as "retrospective-prospective" studies.

One of the meanings of prospective versus retrospective has to do with the time period over which the data were recorded in relation to the time the decision was made to do the study. In this sense, retrospective studies involve a decision to carry out an investigation with observations that have been recorded in the past. In contrast, prospective studies involve the collection of observations after the decision is made to carry out the investigation.

The other meaning of prospective versus retrospective studies is related not to the time sequence of the observations and the decision to do the study but, rather, to the time sequence of observations of study variables and the occurrence of disease. In this sense, prospective studies are analogous to incidence studies, and retrospective studies are analogous to prevalence, or case-control, studies. Prospective or incidence studies measure characteristics and wait for disease to develop, while retrospective or prevalence studies measure the characteristics in persons already diseased.

It is strongly suggested that this second set of definitions be discarded, since better terms are available, as noted. The advantages and disadvantages of prevalence, incidence, and case-control studies will be discussed in Chaps. 6, 7, and 8. The following discussion of prospective versus retrospective studies will consider only the first pair of definitions, relating to when the data were collected.

In prospective studies the investigator can plan and control the methods for making and recording observations, keeping in mind their purpose. In retrospective studies the already-recorded data may have been collected for an entirely unrelated purpose. Therefore these data may well be incomplete and recorded in a manner not appropriate for the present study.

Consequently, there often are severe problems involved in retrospective studies. Consider a study of changes in the outcome of treatment of congestive heart failure in a particular hospital over a period of several years. In carrying out a retrospective study, the investigator would be plagued by the fact that the criteria for the diagnosis of congestive heart failure vary over the years and vary from doctor to doctor. The recent advent of central venous pressure measurements may have improved the ability to diagnose the condition. Cases diagnosed many years ago may differ in character and severity from those diagnosed last year. Therefore observed changes in outcome may be related more to differences in initial severity than to the effects of treatment. If one of the criteria for improvement were weight loss, the investigator would find, to his frustration, that admission and discharge weights were not recorded for many patients over the years, ruling them out of this aspect of the study.

If this study were carried out prospectively, the investigator could initially establish criteria for the diagnosis of congestive heart failure and set up objective measures of severity and improvement. In addition, he could establish procedures to ensure that all the needed measurements were made uniformly on all patients. Thus, the superiority of a prospective study of this question is obvious.

Not all retrospective data need be of poor quality. If we again consider retrospective studies using hospital charts, a variety of data come to mind that would probably have been recorded accurately and consistently. Examples are time of admission, number of days spent in the hospital, sex of the patient, whether the patient died, and whether he received any blood transfusions.

REFERENCE

MacMahon, B., and T. F. Pugh, *Epidemiology: Principles and Methods.* (Boston: Little, Brown, 1970), Chap. 3.

Chapter 5

Descriptive Studies

Descriptive epidemiologic studies reveal the patterns of disease occurrence in human populations. They provide general observations concerning the relationship of disease to basic characteristics. These characteristics include such personal items as age, sex, race, occupation, and social class. Also of great importance are geographic location and time of occurrence of disease. Thus, the major characteristics of interest in descriptive epidemiology may be summarized under the categories: person, place, and time.

At first glance, the goal of describing disease occurrence in this way may seem trivial and not worthy of the efforts of medical scientists. However, such studies are of fundamental importance and serve a variety of purposes—chiefly:

1 Alerting the medical community as to what types of persons (e.g., young or old, male or female, "white collar" workers or "blue collar" workers) are most likely to be affected by a disease, where

the disease will occur, and when. This information is of great value to the physician in making a diagnosis, even though he may not be aware that he is using it.

2   Assisting in the rational planning of health- and medical-care facilities (e.g., number of coronary-care-unit beds needed for the cases of myocardial infarction in a particular community).

3   Providing clues to disease etiology and questions or hypotheses for further fruitful study (e.g., low prevalence of tooth decay in certain areas in the United States suggested further studies concerning the value of fluoride in drinking water).

PERSON

Basic demographic and social characteristics of persons constitute the attributes of greatest concern. Among these characteristics are age, sex, race or ethnic group, marital status, social class or socioeconomic status, religion, and occupation.

Age

Age is one of the most important factors in disease occurrence. Some diseases occur almost exclusively in one particular age group, such as hypertrophic pyloric stenosis in young infants or carcinoma of the prostate in the elderly. Other diseases occur over a much wider age span, but tend to be more prevalent at certain ages than others.

The time of life at which an infectious disease predominates is influenced by such factors as the degree of exposure to the agent at various ages, variations in susceptibility with age, and the duration of the immunity developed after infection. The influence of age-related exposure and duration of immunity is illustrated by the contrast between the single occurrence of chicken pox almost exclusively in young children and the repeated occurrence of gonorrhea, predominantly in adolescents and young adults. Chicken pox is readily transmitted among children playing together or gathering in classrooms, and it produces a lifelong immunity. Gonorrhea is transmitted by sexual contact and results in no immunity.

Many chronic or degenerative diseases such as coronary heart disease and osteoarthritis show a progressive increase in prevalence with increasing age. It is tempting to regard a disease with this age pattern as being due merely to aging itself. It should be remembered, however, that increasing age also marks the passage of time, during which the body is accumulating exposure to harmful environmental influences. For example, the wrinkling and loss of elasticity in skin that we associate with aging can be brought about or accelerated by chronic exposure to sunlight.

Instead of adopting the fatalistic view that a disease is an inevitable consequence of aging, a search for other causative factors should be undertaken. One of the great contributions of epidemiology in the past few decades has been to show that atherosclerosis and its consequences are not due merely to aging, as was previously thought, but that a person's habits and manner of living may contribute importantly to this disease process.

To see how age patterns of disease occurrence lead to clues and hypotheses, note the age trend, reported by Lilienfeld (1956), in the incidence of breast cancer among single and married women in New York State (Fig. 5-1). The steady geometric (note the logarithmic scale) increase in incidence with age diminishes sharply in the forties with a lesser continuing increase in the older years. The reduction in the forties of the rate of increase with age suggested the hypothesis that the hormonal changes of the menopause tend to decrease susceptibility to breast cancer. This hypothesis continues to be of great interest to scientists studying the causes of breast cancer.

Current and Cohort Age Tabulations   The tabulation of disease rates in relation to age at one particular time, as in Fig. 5-1, is known as a *current*, or *cross-sectional*, presentation. This shows disease rates as they are occurring simultaneously in different age groups; thus, different people are involved in each age group. The other way to tabulate and analyze age relationships is in terms of *cohorts*. A cohort is a specific group of people, identified at one period of time and followed up as they pass through different ages during part or all of their life-span.

The results of cross-sectional and cohort age analysis can differ

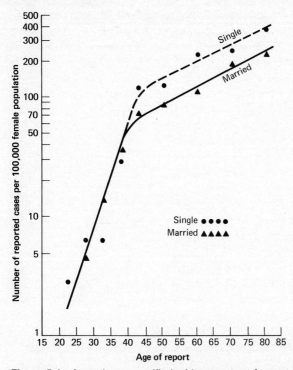

Figure 5-1 Annual age-specific incidence rates of reported cases of female breast cancer, by marital status, New York State exclusive of New York City, 1949. *(Reproduced, by permission, from Lilienfeld, 1956.)*

to a surprising degree, and either approach may be more appropriate for a particular problem. In a classic study, Frost (1939) compared cross-sectional and cohort age analyses of tuberculosis death rates in Massachusetts. Fig. 5-2 shows the cross-sectional curves for males in the years 1880, 1910, and 1930. First of all, note that at all ages the mortality rates decreased between 1880 and 1930. Also, observe that the shapes of the age curves were changing. The 1930 curve was of particular concern to public health workers in the 1930's because it showed tuberculosis mortality rates rising with age

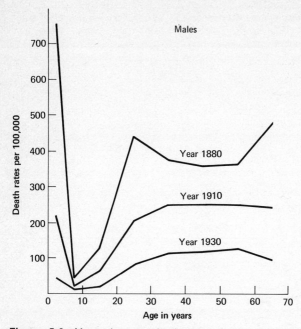

Figure 5-2 Massachusetts death rates from tuberculosis—all forms—by age, 1880, 1910, 1930. *(Reproduced, by permission, from Frost, 1939.)*

in adult life, reaching a maximum between age 50 and 60. This new age pattern of susceptibility to death from tuberculosis was thought possibly to be due to the failure of many individuals to become infected and acquire immunity during youth.

The matter was clarified, however, by a cohort analysis, shown in Fig. 5-3. Each curve represents the cohort of persons born in the 10-year period leading up to and including the year shown above the curve (e.g., 1870 cohort included individuals born from 1861–1870). In this cohort analysis it is apparent that each group experienced its maximum adult risk of tuberculosis death during the age decade of the twenties with subsequent decline in risk with age. Thus, for any particular group of adults, there was no increase in susceptibility with age, after all. The reason that, in 1930, persons in their fifties had higher death rates than younger persons was because they belonged to the 1880 cohort, which experienced a greater exposure to tuberculosis than any of the succeeding cohorts.

Note that the frequently quoted calculations of average life expectancy are determined essentially on a cross-sectional rather than a cohort basis, using what are known as "life tables" (Hill, 1971). The presently observed annual mortality rates for each year of age are applied successively to a hypothetical population beginning either at birth or at some other starting point. It is assumed that as this hypothetical population ages, year by year, it will experience the same mortality rates for each year of life as are now observed in the current population at each age. Actually, the cohort of persons born now may be exposed to different risks of death as they go through

Figure 5-3 Massachusetts death rates from tuberculosis—all forms—by age, in successive 10-year cohorts. *(Reproduced, by permission, from Frost, 1939.)*

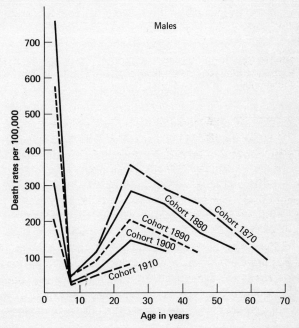

various age periods of life than are experienced by persons who are *now* in those age periods.

Sex

Some diseases occur more frequently in males, others, more frequently in females. If sex-linked inheritance can be excluded, a sex difference in disease incidence initially brings to mind the possibility of hormonal or reproductive factors that either predispose or protect. For example the greater occurrence of coronary heart disease in young men than in young women cannot be explained entirely by sex differences in the so-called coronary risk factors such as blood lipid concentrations, blood pressure, cigarette smoking, diabetes mellitus, and obesity. There may be some important hormonal factor that contributes to the male-female difference—perhaps protection of the female by estrogens before menopause. Similarly, the greater prevalence of gallstones in women than in men is probably attributable, in part, to the effects of repeated pregnancies and, in addition, to hormonal effects on bile composition.

But men and women differ in many other ways, including habits, social relationships, environmental exposures, and other aspects of day-to-day living. The higher male prevalence of cirrhosis of the liver and chronic bronchitis are at least partly related to the fact that, on the average, men currently drink more alcohol and smoke more cigarettes than women.

Sex differences in disease occurrence are important descriptive findings and often suggest avenues for further research. No disease can be considered to have a well-understood etiology if it manifests a male or female predominance which is not explained.

Race

Racial differences in disease prevalence have often been noted. In the case of some diseases (e.g., black-white differences in sickle-cell anemia and skin cancer), the differences are genetically determined. With other diseases, the explanation may not be so simple, especially when racial differences are accompanied by differences in socioeconomic status.

A case in point is the higher prevalence of hypertension and its complications in blacks than in whites in the United States. Suggested explanations have included (1) increased genetic susceptibility in blacks, (2) increased emotional stress in blacks due to racial discrimination, (3) lower average socioeconomic levels in blacks (since in whites the prevalence of hypertension is higher in lower socioeconomic groups), and (4) less access for blacks to good medical care (Howard and Holman, 1970). It may eventually be shown that some or all of these mechanisms are involved.

Marital Status

Marital status is another important descriptive variable. Married persons have lower mortality rates than single persons, including both overall mortality and mortality from most specific diseases. Whether the married state provides health benefits or whether characteristics favoring long life also predispose to marriage has not been decided.

Of great interest in studies of cancer etiology has been the contrast between cancer of the breast and cancer of the uterine cervix in their relation to marital status. Breast cancer is more apt to develop in single women or women who marry late in life, while cervical cancer is associated with early marriage. Further studies stemming, in part, from these observations suggest that cervical cancer is associated with coital activity at an early age and that having a first pregnancy at an early age may help protect a woman from breast cancer.

The data regarding the relationship of breast cancer incidence to age (see Fig. 5-1) also revealed a higher incidence in single women than in married women in their forties and later age decades. Lilienfeld suggested the hypothesis that early artificial or surgical menopause, occurring more often in married than in single women, might be protective against breast cancer. This hypothesis received some confirmation in an analytic case-control study in which it was found that (1) women with breast cancer less often gave a history of artificial menopause than did control subjects, and (2) married women more often gave a history of artificial menopause than did single women.

Socioeconomic Status

Socioeconomic status or social class is a somewhat nebulous concept, but it can be measured fairly conveniently by the occupation or income of the family head, by his or her educational level, or by residence, in terms of the value and amenities of the home or dwelling unit. The British have used occupation to define five social classes—I. Professional, II. Intermediate, III. Skilled, IV. Partly Skilled, and V. Unskilled. Using this classification system, the Registrar General for England and Wales has provided descriptive data relating social class to a variety of conditions.

As mentioned in our discussion of hypertension, many diseases show a distinct social class gradient, with higher rates in the lower socioeconomic classes. Included are rheumatic heart disease, chronic bronchitis, tuberculosis, stomach ulcer, stomach cancer, and nutritional-deficiency diseases.

On the other hand, low socioeconomic status appears to confer protection against some diseases. In the series of annual poliomyelitis epidemics that began in 1947, the higher social classes were the most severely affected. It is believed that in economically disadvantaged groups, poor sanitary conditions had resulted in widespread subclinical infection in the first few years of life, resulting in immunity. When "higher" living standards prevent this early infection, acquiring poliomyelitis later in childhood is more likely to cause paralytic disease.

A marked socioeconomic gradient in infant mortality has long been noted. Table 5-1 shows social class and rates of infant mortality (at age under one year) per 1,000 live births in England and Wales during two time periods, 1930–1932 and 1949–1953. Note that even though there was a marked improvement by the later time period, Social Class V still had over twice the infant mortality rate observed in Social Class I. Infant mortality rates have often been used as an index both of living standards and of availability of medical services in comparing nations or areas within a nation.

PLACE

Where disease occurs is a matter of great importance. Comparison of disease rates in different places may provide obvious clues to

Table 5-1 Infant Mortality Rates in England and Wales as Related to Social Class during Two Time Periods, 1930–1932 and 1949–1953

Social class	Infant mortality rates*	
	1930–1932	1949–1953
I	32.7	18.7
II	45.0	21.6
III	57.6	28.6
IV	66.8	33.8
V	77.1	40.8
All classes	61.6	29.5

*Deaths of infants under one year old per 1,000 live births. Registrar General's data, Taylor and Knowelden (1964).

etiology or serve as a stimulus to further fruitful investigation. The places of concern may be as large as a continent or as small as part of a room. As illustrative examples, descriptive findings will be presented from international comparisons, comparisons of regions within the United States and Canada, and comparisons of areas in a city.

International Comparisons

Because of the problems regarding the validity of mortality statistics, described in Chap. 3, it is difficult to take seriously small differences among nations in mortality rates for specific diseases. However, it is also difficult to explain away very large differences as due to artifact—that is, where the death rate for a disease in one country is two or three times as large as the death rate in another. Large differences are particularly impressive when both countries are known to have reasonably good vital statistics systems.

The Unique Position of Japan Ranking the disease-specific mortality rates of various nations has revealed Japan to be among the highest nations for some diseases and among the lowest for others. Table 5-2 shows some age-adjusted or age-specific mortality rates for stomach cancer, colon cancer, breast cancer, cerebrovascular disease (primarily strokes), and coronary heart disease. Note that among the nations studied, Japan is the highest ranking country for stomach cancer and cerebrovascular disease and the lowest ranking for breast cancer, colon cancer, and coronary heart disease.

Because of Japan's unique position among nations regarding these diseases, consideration of the mode of life in Japan has suggested a number of questions and hypotheses for further study. The relatively frequent practice and long duration of breast feeding of infants in Japan has raised the question of whether lactation may diminish the risk of developing breast cancer. The traditional Japanese diet has come under considerable scrutiny in hopes of finding predisposing factors for stomach cancer and protective factors for colon cancer. Also, the low fat intake in Japan has been thought responsible for the low average serum-cholesterol levels observed there and the low incidence of coronary heart disease. Although some portion of the high cerebrovascular death rate may be due to a known tendency of Japanese to attribute any sudden death to a cerebral hemorrhage, the high salt intake of Japanese has come under suspicion as a possible predisposing factor for hypertension and stroke.

Many traditional practices in Japan are now changing, and it will be of considerable interest to learn whether disease rates will change in ways that are consistent with the above hypotheses. Already, the migration of Japanese to places where they adopt new eating and living habits has permitted comparative studies aimed at identifying environmental factors that predispose to disease. Gordon (1957) compared mortality rates for Japanese in Japan, Hawaii, and the United States mainland and found contrasting trends for cerebrovascular disease and for coronary heart disease. Cerebrovascular disease mortality rates in both sexes decreased, and coronary mortality rates in men increased from Japan to Hawaii to the United States mainland. This suggested that as Japanese were adopting "the American way of life," their susceptibility to the two diseases in question was moving in the direction of that found in other Americans. (The assumption that migrants are genetically similar to those who remain in their native land should always be viewed with caution.) In order to explore in detail the reasons for the

Table 5-2 Ranking of Death Rates of Various Countries, from Highest to Lowest*

Rank	Stomach cancer, males, 1964–1965	Colon cancer (except rectum), males, 1964–1965	Breast cancer, females, 1964–1965	Cerebrovascular disease, males, ages 65–74, 1964	Coronary heart disease, males, ages 45–54, 1964
1	Japan (69)	Scotland (16)	Netherlands (26)	Japan (1,680)	Finland (442)
2	Chile (58)	Denmark (14)	England & Wales (24)	Scotland (901)	Scotland (358)
3	Austria (42)	U.S.A.—white (14)	Denmark (24)	Finland (751)	U.S.A. (354)
4	Finland (40)	Canada (13)	Scotland (24)	West Germany (750)	Australia (324)
5	West Germany (37)	New Zealand (13)	Canada (23)	Italy (708)	Northern Ireland (324)
6	Italy (34)	Northern Ireland (13)	New Zealand (23)	Hungary (706)	Canada (311)
7	Portugal (33)	Ireland (13)	South Africa (23)	Austria (663)	New Zealand (293)
8	Netherlands (28)	Australia (12)	Northern Ireland (22)	Northern Ireland (656)	England & Wales (245)
9	Belgium (27)	Belgium (12)	U.S.A.—white (22)	Israel (614)	Israel (214)
10	Switzerland (26)	England & Wales (12)	Switzerland (22)	England & Wales (612)	West Germany (183)
11	Norway (26)	France (12)	Ireland (22)	Australia (611)	Denmark (181)
12	Scotland (25)	Switzerland (11)	Belgium (21)	Czechoslovakia (560)	Norway (164)
13	South Africa (25)	U.S.A.—nonwhite (11)	Israel (21)	Switzerland (530)	Netherlands (162)
14	Ireland (24)	Netherlands (11)	U.S.A.—nonwhite (20)	France (528)	Austria (159)
15	England & Wales (23)	South Africa (11)	Australia (19)	U.S.A. (495)	Belgium (159)
16	Sweden (22)	Austria (10)	Sweden (19)	Norway (492)	Czechoslovakia (151)
17	Northern Ireland (22)	West Germany (10)	West Germany (18)	Denmark (478)	Hungary (147)
18	Denmark (22)	Sweden (10)	Austria (17)	New Zealand (475)	Switzerland (134)
19	France (21)	Norway (8)	Norway (17)	Netherlands (416)	Italy (133)
20	Israel (18)	Italy (8)	France (16)	Canada (414)	Venezuela (131)
21	U.S.A.—nonwhite (18)	Portugal (8)	Italy (16)	Sweden (394)	Sweden (125)
22	Canada (18)	Israel (7)	Finland (14)	Belgium (334)	France (74)
23	New Zealand (17)	Finland (5)	Portugal (13)	Venezuela (281)	Japan (51)
24	Australia (15)	Chile (4)	Chile (9)		
25	U.S.A.—white (9)	Japan (3)	Japan (4)		

*Death rates per 100,000 shown in parentheses (rounded from the original).

Sources: Stomach, colon, and breast cancer: Segi et al. (1969); cerebrovascular and coronary heart disease: World Health Organization (1967).

above geographic trends in cerebrovascular and coronary disease, parallel data collection methods have been established in three on-going epidemiologic studies of Japanese, located in Hiroshima, Japan; Honolulu, Hawaii; and in the San Francisco Bay area (Belsky et al., 1971).

Comparisons of Regions within Countries

The availability of mortality statistics for states and finer geographic subdivisions in the United States and other nations has permitted the discovery of interesting place-to-place variations in disease occurrence. Differences in mortality rates between urban and rural areas are a common finding. The higher mortality from lung cancer in cities than in farming areas is consistent with an etiologic role of either cigarette smoking or air pollution, since both are more common in cities.

The North-to-South Gradient of Multiple Sclerosis Geographic variation within nations may take the form of a distinct north-to-south gradient, which suggests that climate or other factors related to latitude may be involved. An example is the finding in the United States and Canada of generally higher mortality rates for multiple sclerosis the farther north one looks (Fig. 5-4). Confirmation of the north-to-south trend also comes from other nations and from prevalence rates found in several cities (Fig. 5-5). While hypotheses abound, to date no one has convincingly explained this geographic distribution of multiple sclerosis (Alter, 1968).

Areas within a City

When studying disease occurrence within a city, it is often desirable to plot the occurrence of disease in each census tract, since information about other characteristics of persons in each tract is available.

Rheumatic Fever in Baltimore Figure 5-7 from Gordis et al. (1969) shows the distribution in Baltimore census tracts of the homes of hospitalized rheumatic fever cases in 1960–1964. Most of

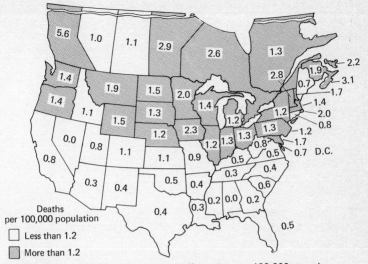

Figure 5-4 Multiple sclerosis mortality rates per 100,000 population in the U.S. states and in Canadian provinces. *(Reproduced, by permission, from Alter, 1968, adapted from Limburg, 1950.)*

Figure 5-5 Multiple sclerosis prevalence rates in cities of the United States and Canada. *(Reproduced, by permission, from Alter, 1968.)*

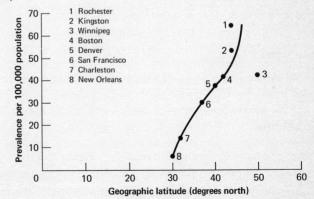

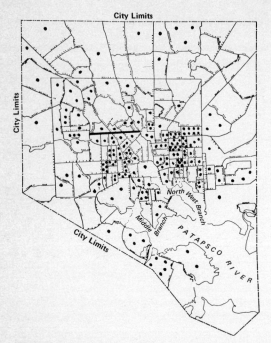

Figure 5-6 Residence distribution of hospitalized rheumatic fever patients, Baltimore 1960–1964. Heavy line shows North Avenue. Each dot represents one patient. *(Reproduced, by permission, from Gordis et al., 1969.)*

the cases occurred in two clusters on either side of the central business district—in the low-income area south of North Avenue, which is shown by a heavy line. Naturally, we cannot form a judgment based only on the "numerator" cases but must relate these to the "denominator" populations in each tract to develop rates.

Thus, annual incidence rates were calculated for groups of census tracts in this area and ranged as high as 40.2 per 100,000. In contrast, the incidence rate for the entire city was only 15.6 per 100,000.

Studying the high and low incidence areas further revealed that nonwhite children suffered a higher incidence of rheumatic fever than did whites. Only among whites was higher socioeconomic status related to lower incidence of rheumatic fever. When housing characteristics were examined, the degree of crowding was the variable that was most closely related to rheumatic fever occurrence. The authors emphasized the importance of socioeconomic conditions in this disease and showed that the higher incidence in nonwhites might have been due to the crowded living conditions in which most Baltimore nonwhites lived.

TIME

The pattern of disease occurrence in time is often an extremely informative descriptive characteristic. A great variety of time trends may be found in the literature; these involve simple increases or decreases of disease incidence, or more complex combinations of these changes in time. To provide an introduction to this interesting subject, a few examples of short-term, periodic, and long-term trends will be described.

Short-term Increases and Decreases in Disease Incidence

Short-term changes are those increases or decreases in disease incidence that are measured in hours, days, weeks, or months. These are most often observed in the study of epidemics of infectious disease, as will be illustrated below. However, important short-term trends also have been noted in the occurrence of symptoms of, or even deaths due to, chronic noninfectious disease, in relation to both natural phenomena such as heat waves and man-made stresses such as marked increases in air pollution.

Epidemics An *epidemic*, or *outbreak*, is the occurrence of a disease in members of a defined population clearly in excess of the number of cases usually or normally found in *that* population. In investigating epidemics, a careful tabulation of the distribution of disease-onset times of the affected members of the population, in terms either of counts of cases or incidence ("attack") rates, may be very helpful in determining the initiating causes and mechanism of spread.

For a thorough discussion of the propagation of epidemics the reader is referred to Sartwell (1965). A few basic principles should be mentioned, however, before we consider some examples of time patterns. Epidemics only affect susceptible members of the population, of which there may be many or few. Others in the population are immune due to antibodies related to previous disease occurrence, immunization, or passive transfer from mother to infant. Still others may be resistant due to other inherent factors. After a person is exposed to the disease-causing agent, there is an incubation period until the disease first appears. Susceptible persons may also develop inapparent infections, in which no symptoms or signs become evident. The infectious agent may leave the host during the communicable period, which varies in timing and duration from one disease to the next.

Infections are transmitted from one person to another in a variety of ways: by direct personal contact, by touching contaminated objects, or by droplets spraying from one person to another close by, as during talking or sneezing. Evaporation of such droplets may yield "droplet nuclei" which, like certain disease-carrying dusts, may remain airborne for longer periods and travel longer distances. Other modes of transmission include vehicles such as certain foods or water, and *vectors* such as arthropods which carry the infectious agent.

The infection is usually introduced into the population directly or indirectly by one or more persons. If there is a sufficient proportion of susceptibles and the infection spreads rapidly enough, the disease will show a trend of increasing incidence through time to a maximum, followed by a fairly steady diminution until the disease disappears completely or almost completely. The decrease is largely due to the fact that the population begins to run out of susceptible individuals as those who were previously susceptible acquire the disease and become immune. As susceptibles become increasingly scarce, the infectious agent, no matter how well and how rapidly transmitted, finds less and less fertile soil in which to grow, so to speak. The rise through time from a negligible incidence rate to a maximum followed by a fall to low levels again appears graphically as a simple epidemic curve, usually but not always involving short-term trends involving days, weeks, or months.

Fig. 5-7 shows an epidemic of measles (rubeola) that occurred

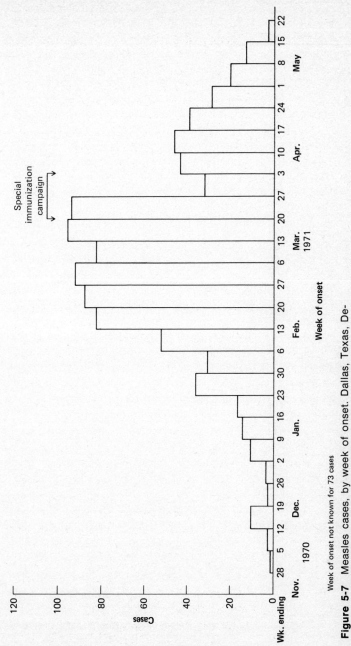

Week of onset not known for 73 cases

Figure 5-7 Measles cases, by week of onset. Dallas, Texas, December 1, 1970–May 22, 1971. *(Reproduced, by permission, from Luby et al., 1971.)*

among children in Dallas, Texas from late 1970 almost to the middle of 1971 (Luby et al., 1971). By May 1971 there were 1,071 reported cases. The histogram displaying the epidemic's time sequence is of special interest because it shows an abrupt drop after the apparent peak of the epidemic was reached at the end of March. During the 2-week period in which the abrupt fall in case counts began, a special immunization campaign for children was carried out. Although alternative explanations should be considered, it appears that the campaign was helpful in controlling the epidemic by sharply reducing the number of susceptible individuals in the population.

The observed time pattern of an epidemic may provide a strong indication of the mode of initiation and spread. Figs. 5-8 and 5-9 show two different outbreaks of the same disease, infectious hepatitis. Fig. 5-8 depicts the number of cases, by *week* of onset, in an epidemic occurring in Barren County, Kentucky, lasting from June 1970 through April 1971. Fig. 5-9 is drawn on a different time scale and shows the number of cases, by *day* of onset, in an epidemic that occurred in Orange County, California, between August 21, 1971 and September 13, 1971.

The essential distinction between the two epidemics is their duration, particularly in relation to the known incubation period of this disease, which ranges from 15 to 50 days and is commonly about 25 days.

Although the communicable period for this disease has not been clearly defined, the clustering of the Orange County cases within such a narrow time interval—the great bulk appearing within 9 days and all within 24 days—suggested that the outbreak resulted from a "point source," that is, a single common exposure to the virus. With an incubation period measured in weeks, person-to-person spread among the group of cases could not have been a significant factor in an epidemic that ended so soon after it started.

In contrast, the bulk of the Barren County cases occurred over an interval of 4 months, and the total epidemic lasted for 10 months, so there was ample time for direct person-to-person spread. This mode of transmission, however, would not be the only possible mechanism consistent with a hepatitis epidemic of this duration. Prolonged exposure of a population to a contaminated food or water supply could also result in a long-lasting epidemic. However, no such mechanism could be incriminated in Barren County.

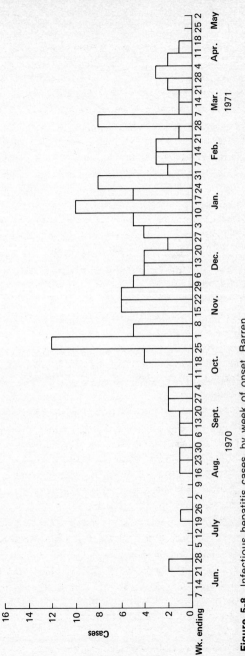

Figure 5-8 Infectious hepatitis cases, by week of onset, Barren County, Kentucky, June, 1970–April, 1971. *(Reproduced, by permission, from Carman et al., 1971.)*

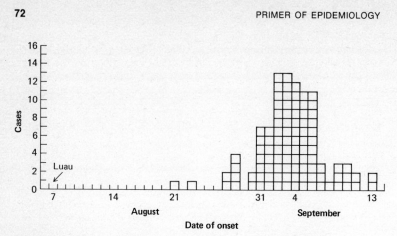

Figure 5-9 Cases of infectious hepatitis in individuals attending luau, by day of onset, Orange County, California, 1971. (Date of onset for one case undetermined.) *(Reproduced, by permission, from Philp et al., 1972).*

Further investigation of each epidemic revealed quite interesting information. In Barren County, most of the 118 cases occurred in children attending two elementary schools. The first observed case in June occurred in a boy whose parents frequently baby-sat for other children in the area. Among the children exposed to his parents was a seven-year-old boy who was the first hepatitis case at one of the schools. The seven-year-old's illness began on September 26. All but one of the cases involving children in that school and their families could be traced directly or indirectly to contact with the seven-year-old. Similarly, at the other school the first illness occurred in a nine-year-old girl on September 21. It was not determined how she became infected but she spread the disease to a total of 34 persons via 5 children with whom she had contact (Carman et al., 1971).

In Orange County almost all the 99 cases were members of a private sailing club. The only time all the cases were together during the prior year was at a club luau at a remote island off the California coast on August 7. One clue to the vehicle of infection was found in the age distribution of incidence. The attack rate was 6 percent in persons under age 15 and was 62 percent in persons age 15 and over.

Detailed analysis of suspect foods revealed only one item regarding which *all* persons *not* consuming it remained free of the disease. This was a mai-tai punch. Sizable proportions of persons *not* eating each of the other foods did become ill, which tends to exonerate these other food items. The description of the food-handling situation at the luau by Philp and his associates (1972) clearly shows how the mai-tai could have served as the vehicle for the fecal-oral transmission of the hepatitis virus.

All food and beverages were brought to the island by boat. Commercial bottled water for drinking was imported. Little attention, however, was paid to food-handling practices. The only water for handwashing was a single water tap located 85 yards beyond the luau site and 35 yards beyond the two privies available to the group. Handwashing was a rare event. Foods were cooked in an earthen pit for 6 hours to the point of disintegration. Unwashed papaya, pineapple, and oranges were peeled and cut for a fruit mix. Mai-tai punch was prepared from the cut fruits, unwashed fresh strawberries, instant tea, canned pineapple juice, canned lemon-lime drink, bottled water, club soda, and rum. All were mixed in a new plastic garbage can. The punch was served from a 3-tiered fountain made with fiberglass bowls suspended over the garbage can reservoir. Punch was pumped from the can to the top of the fountain, where it flowed over the fiberglass tiers back down into the garbage can. Persons who drank punch filled their cups under one of the streams as it cascaded from one bowl to the next. Many reported punch running over their hands and back into the punch reservoir. Due to the presence of pieces of fruit, particularly strawberries, the pump which forced the punch to the top of the fountain plugged frequently and was unplugged by one or more persons reaching into the bottom of the garbage can and pulling fruit pieces out of the pump. Persons who unclogged the pump also reported sand at the bottom of the can.

Recurrent or Periodic Time Trends

The incidence of certain diseases shows regular recurring increases and decreases. This regular pattern may exhibit cycles which last several years. Many cycles occur annually and represent seasonal variation in disease occurrence. Seasonal variation is a well-known characteristic for many infectious diseases and is usually based on characteristics of the infectious agent itself, the life pattern of its vector or other animal hosts, or changes in the likelihood of person-to-person spread. For example, waterborne gastrointestinal infections often exhibit a peak occurrence in the later summer months when recreational swimming and other factors facilitate their transmission. On the other hand upper respiratory infections frequently show a seasonal rise in or near winter, aided by the concentration of people indoors where virus-containing airborne droplets are readily exchanged.

Shorter-term periodic variations have also been observed. For example, death rates from automobile accidents show weekly cycles with the highest rates occurring on weekends, particularly Saturdays. To date there are no available statistics on the number of passenger-miles driven on each day of the week. Thus it is not possible to state whether the weekend increase in deaths is due merely to an increased exposure of the population to the moving automobile or whether the risk of death per passenger-mile actually increases, possibly due to such factors as more reckless driving or more alcohol consumption on weekends.

Long-term or Secular Trends

Some diseases exhibit a progressive increase or decrease in occurrence that is manifested over years or decades. These long-term time trends are often referred to as *secular* trends.

Figure 5-10 shows the mortality rates in United States males of several leading types of cancer, from 1930 to 1968. A marked secular increase in mortality from lung cancer has occurred, representing about a fifteenfold increase in 1967 as compared to 1930. This increase is believed to be due largely to an increase in the proportion of men who smoked cigarettes. Fig. 5-10 also shows a marked downward trend in stomach cancer mortality. This improvement has not been explained but remains gratifying, nonetheless.

As has been discussed, when a marked increase in incidence occurs in a short period of time, it is quite apparent to the medical community and is referred to as an epidemic, an emotionally loaded

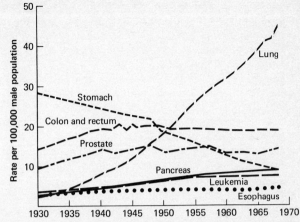

Figure 5-10 Age-adjusted male cancer death rates, by site, United States, 1930–1968. *(Reproduced, by permission, from Silverberg and Holleb, 1972. Data from the U.S. National Vital Statistics Division and Bureau of the Census.)*

term that spurs prompt action. Long-term trends are barely perceptible and might go unnoticed were it not for the study of vital statistics. It would perhaps be well to label as "epidemics," the long-term increases such as that noted for lung cancer. If this term were applied, more action might be taken to investigate the causes and to institute control measures.

REFERENCES

Alter, M. 1968. Etiologic considerations based on the epidemiology of multiple sclerosis. *Amer. J. Epidemiology*, 88:318–332.

Belsky, J. L., A. Kagan, and S. L. Syme. 1971. Epidemiologic studies of coronary heart disease and stroke in Japanese men living in Japan, Hawaii, and California. Research Plan. *Atomic Bomb Casualty Comm. Tech. Rep.*, 12–71.

Carman, M., W. B. Guerrant, and C. Hernandez. 1971. Infectious hepatitis—Kentucky. *Center for Disease Control: Morbidity and Mortality Weekly Report.* 20:136–137.

Frost, W. H. 1939. The age selection of mortality from tuberculosis in successive decades. *Amer. J. Hyg.* 30:91–96.

Gordis, L., A. Lilienfeld, and R. Rodriguez. 1969. Studies in the epidemiology and preventability of rheumatic fever: I. Demographic factors and the incidence of acute attacks, and II. Socio-economic factors and the incidence of acute attacks. *J. Chron. Dis.* 21:645–666.

Gordon, T. 1957. Mortality experience among the Japanese in the United States, Hawaii and Japan. *Public Health Reports* 72:543–553.

Hill, A. B., *Principles of Medical Statistics.* (London: Oxford University Press, 1971), pp. 220–228.

Howard, J., and B. L. Holman. 1970. The effects of race and occupation on hypertension mortality. *Milbank Memorial Fund Quarterly* 48:263–296.

Lilienfeld, A. M. 1956. The relationship of cancer of the female breast to artificial menopause and marital status. *Cancer,* 9:927–934.

Limburg, C. C. 1950. Geographic distribution of multiple sclerosis and its estimated prevalence in the United States. *Proceedings of the Association for Research in Nervous and Mental Diseases,* 28:15–24, Baltimore: Williams and Wilkins.

Luby, J. P., H. J. Dewlett, and M. S. Dickerson. 1971. Measles—Dallas, Texas. *Center for Disease Control: Morbidity and Mortality Weekly Report,* 20:191–192.

Philp, J. R., T. P. Hamilton, T. J. Albert, R. S. Stone, C. F. Pait, R. R. Roberto, N. J. Fiumara, A. R. Hinman, and C. Friedmann. 1972. Hepatitis A Outbreak, Orange County, Calif. *Center for Disease Control: Hepatitis Surveillance,* Report No. 35, pp. 12–13. See also *Amer. J. Epidemiology* 97:50–54, 1973.

Sartwell, P. E., (Ed.): *Maxcy-Rosenow Preventive Medicine and Public Health, Ninth Edition.* (New York: Appleton-Century-Crofts, 1965), Chap. 4.

Segi, M., M. Kurihara, and T. Matsuyama, *Cancer Mortality for Selected Sites in 24 Countries. No. 5 (1964–1965).* Department of Public Health, Tohoku University School of Medicine. Sendai, Japan, 1969.

Silverberg, E., and A. I. Holleb. 1972. Cancer statistics, 1972. *Ca–A Cancer Journal for Clinicians,* 22:2–20.

Taylor, I., and J. Knowelden, *Principles of Epidemiology.* (Boston: Little, Brown, 1964), Chaps. 6, 7 (infectious epidemics); Chap. 12, pp. 318–321 (social class).

World Health Organization: 1967. Mortality statistics: cardiovascular diseases, annual statistics, 1955–1964, by sex and age. *Epidemiological Vital Statistics Reports,* 20:535–710.

Chapter 6

Prevalence Studies

In going beyond descriptive observations to delve more deeply into disease etiology, there are, as defined in Chap. 4, three basic types of observational investigations:

1 Prevalence or cross-sectional studies
2 Case-control studies
3 Incidence or cohort studies

These will be discussed in greater detail here and in the next two chapters. As will be seen, prevalence studies are, conceptually, quite straightforward, and provide a good basis for subsequent consideration and comparison of the other two study types.

How Prevalence Studies Are Carried Out

   Initial Steps   The question(s) for study must be clearly defined in terms of the relationship between some possible predisposing factor(s) and the disease under investigation. Then a suitable study population is identified. If this population is small enough to be studied using the human and financial resources available (e.g., students in a school, adults in a small town), the entire population can be included. If the target population is too large (e.g., children in the United States, men in a large city), then a representative sample is selected.

Sampling Methods for selecting an appropriate sample constitute an important and well-developed field of statistical study, and cannot be dealt with comprehensively in this book. The reader should be familiar with a few basic types of samples, since sampling may be necessary in any type of epidemiologic study. For a more complete discussion the reader is referred to Hansen et al. (1953) and Hill (1971).

The most elementary kind of sample is a *simple random sample* in which each person has an equal chance of being selected directly out of the entire population. One way to carry out this procedure is to assign each person a number, starting with 1, 2, 3, and so on. Then, numbers are selected at random, usually from a table of random numbers (see Arkin and Colton, 1963), until the desired sample size is attained.

A *stratified random sample* involves dividing the population into distinct subgroups according to some important characteristic, such as age or socioeconomic status, and selecting a random sample out of each subgroup. If the proportion of the sample drawn from each of the subgroups, or *strata*, is the same as the proportion of the total population comprised by each stratum (e.g., age group 40–59 comprises 20 percent of the population, and 20 percent of the sample comes from this age stratum), then all strata will be fairly represented with regard to numbers of persons in the sample. This proportionality is often desirable and may simplify data analysis. On the other hand, the investigator may have to take a larger proportion of his study sample out of one or a few sparsely populated strata, in order to make available for study adequate numbers of subjects with certain important characteristics.

A *cluster sample* involves (1) dividing the population into subgroups, or *clusters*, that are not necessarily (and preferably not) homogeneous, as are strata, (2) drawing a random sample of the clusters, and (3) selecting all or a random sample of the persons in each cluster. When each cluster comprises persons in a localized geographic area, such as a county, cluster sampling is especially useful for national surveys. It is obvious that many more persons can be studied for the same cost if they live in a few U.S. counties, than if they are scattered all over the country.

Finally, *systematic samples* involve first deciding what fraction of the population is to be studied—for example, one-half or one-tenth—and listing the population in order, perhaps as in a directory or on a series of index cards. Then, starting at the beginning of the list, every second or every tenth (or whatever interval is dictated by the fraction to be chosen) is selected. In order to sample in this manner, the investigator must be quite sure that the intervals do not correspond with any recurring pattern in the population. Consider what would happen if the population were made up of a series of married couples with the husband always listed first. Picking every fourth person would result in a sample of men only, if one started with the first or third subject, or of women only, if one started with the second or fourth.

Sampling can be done in multiple stages, such as sampling within strata which are, in turn, within clusters. In this manner, sampling can become quite involved and require expert assistance in planning. Experience has also revealed subtle problems and biases that might not occur to the novice. Sampling by households is a good example. If there is no one home when the interviewer arrives, he or she should come back again rather than go to the house next door, because households with a person at home in the daytime tend to differ from those without. Similarly, the first house seen as one approaches a new block should not be routinely called upon, since persons in corner houses tend to differ from those in the middle of the block.

Data Collection   Once the total study population or sample is defined, the necessary data are collected. Presence of disease may be determined in a variety of ways. For example, in a small town, all or almost all the existing cases of a disease can often be found by contacting all the practicing physicians and reviewing hospital records. Or, the disease can be detected by a special examination of all the residents.

The presence of, or exposure to, the possible causative factors under investigation should also be determined by appropriate tests and measurements. For example, in considering the possible role of inhaled factors, degree of cigarette smoking can be determined by interview, and air pollution levels in various places of living or work can be determined by appropriate measuring devices.

Data Analysis   The usual way to tabulate the data in a prevalence study is to subdivide the population according to the suspected predisposing factors being studied and compare the disease prevalence rates in each subgroup. If the relationship of chronic cough to number of cigarettes smoked is to be studied in a group of middle-aged men, then the group may be divided into appropriate smoking categories, such as: none, less than one-half pack per day, one-half pack or more but less than one pack, one pack or more but less than two packs, and two packs or more. The prevalence rate of chronic cough is then determined for each smoking subgroup and the rates in the subgroups are compared. Of course, before the rates are computed, strict criteria must be established for the definition of what constitutes "chronic cough."

Interpretation

In general, the prevalence study will show the presence or absence of a relationship between the study variable(s) and existing disease. *Existing* disease, as contrasted with *developing* disease found in an incidence study, implies a need for caution, since existing cases may not be representative of *all* cases of the disease.

Consider coronary heart disease, for example. One of the important manifestations of coronary heart disease is sudden unexpected death. In a prevalence survey, cases of coronary heart disease showing sudden unexpected death as their first clinical manifestation will be missed because the duration of recognizable disease is so extremely short. It would indeed be remarkable if such a case happened to occur just at the moment the individual was taking the survey examination! From this extreme example it can readily be seen that the shorter the duration of the disease, whether it kills or is cured rapidly, the less chance its victim has of being detected in a one-time prevalence survey. It follows logically, then, that cases of long duration are overrepresented in a prevalence study. The characteristics of these long-duration cases may, on the average, differ in a variety of ways from the characteristics of all cases of the disease being studied.

While we are considering the duration of illness of diseased persons in a prevalence study, it would be worthwhile to digress slightly and point out that there are two basic properties of a disease that are reflected in its prevalence. One is how much disease develops per unit of time, or incidence; the other is how long it lasts, or duration. In fact, under stable conditions, where the incidence and duration of a disease have remained constant over a period of time, the relationship between prevalence, incidence, and duration can be expressed as a simple mathematical equation: Prevalence equals incidence times mean duration ($P = I\bar{d}$). Thus, if any one of the three measures is unknown, it can be computed from the other two, provided that conditions are stable, as mentioned.

Another factor leads to "prevalence cases" being an unrepresentative sample of all cases; that is, if certain types of cases leave the community. Some affected persons may be institutionalized elsewhere or move to another city where there are special facilities for treatment, thus escaping local surveillance procedures.

When interpreting the findings of a prevalence study, care must be taken to avoid assigning an unsubstantiated time sequence to an association between a trait or other factor and the disease. If it is found, for example, that cancer patients exhibit more anxiety or other emotional problems than the unaffected members of the population, it cannot be assumed that the anxiety preceded the cancer. After all, cancer patients may have good reason to be nervous or disturbed. In contrast, there would be no doubt about the cancer being preceded by such traits as eye color, blood type, or maternal exposure to radiation.

Example I: Prevalence Studies of Chronic Respiratory Disease in Berlin, New Hampshire

In 1961, Ferris and Anderson (1962) carried out a prevalence study of chronic respiratory disease in relation to cigarette smoking and air pollution in Berlin, New Hampshire. This industrial town with almost

18,000 inhabitants is located in a valley near the Canadian border and is almost completely surrounded by mountains. The major industry and chief source of air pollution is a paper and pulp mill.

In this study, the investigators planned to diagnose three disease states—chronic bronchitis, bronchial asthma, and irreversible obstructive lung disease—using simple pulmonary function tests and a standardized interview questionnaire about respiratory symptoms. These standardized methods for assessing pulmonary disease, developed and tested in Great Britain and already used in several studies, would permit a comparison of the findings in Berlin, New Hampshire to those in British and other population groups. At that time there was great interest in the apparent disparity in the relative frequency of chronic bronchitis in Great Britain and the United States, and it was believed that differences in diagnostic criteria and fashions might have been at least partially responsible.

The investigators, in cooperation with the local health department, selected the study sample in two stages. First, using the town's tax roll book which listed the adults in alphabetical order, they randomly selected 36 pages (clusters). Second, from the 36 pages they systematically selected every second name of those in the 25–54-year age stratum and all names of persons aged 55–69. Persons aged 70 and over were listed separately in the town records, and a sample of this age stratum was randomly selected.

Before any data were collected, the local physicians and the state Health Department were contacted and the study was publicized by newspaper and radio. The study subjects were invited by letter to take the study examination at a clinic in the Health Department. Failure to respond led to a telephoned invitation, and if this, in turn, failed, the subject was visited at home and, if he agreed, the interview and physiologic testing were carried out there. Through these persistent efforts, over 95 percent of the 1,261 selected subjects were examined, with the only nonparticipants being those who were away from home during the survey and a few who refused.

Respiratory symptoms were elicited by the standardized interview. Smoking habits, occupational exposures, and previous chest illnesses were also assessed in the interview. Forced expiratory volume, both total (FEV) and during the first second ($FEV_{1.0}$), and peak flow were measured with a recording vitalometer.

The presence of disease was defined by strict criteria. For example, the diagnosis of chronic bronchitis required "the report of bringing up phlegm from the chest six times a day on four days a week for three months in a year, for the past three years or more."

Data analysis revealed a greater prevalence of respiratory disease in men than in women. Furthermore, there was a clear relationship of respiratory disease to smoking. For example, in men the age-adjusted prevalence of chronic bronchitis was:

15.0% in those who had never smoked
18.9% in exsmokers
29.8% in smokers of 1–10 cigarettes per day
34.2% in smokers of 11–20 cigarettes per day
42.3% in smokers of 21–30 cigarettes per day
61.1% in smokers of 31–40 cigarettes per day
75.3% in smokers of 41 or more cigarettes per day

The town was divided into three areas with low, intermediate, and high degrees of air pollution, according to independent measurements of air quality. Residence of study subjects in these three areas showed only an equivocal relationship to respiratory disease. However, if only nonsmokers were considered, it appeared that among men, chronic bronchitis was more apt to be found in residential areas having greater air pollution.

The planned United States–British comparison was later reported by Reid et al. (1964). The findings in Berlin, New Hampshire were compared with those derived from a random sample of urban and rural dwelling adults in Britain examined in a comparable fashion. It was found that the British exceeded the Americans very little in the prevalence of simple chronic bronchitis, characterized by chronic cough and sputum production. However, bronchitis complicated with shortness of breath and repeated acute illnesses was more prevalent in Britain, particularly in urban men.

The prevalence survey in Berlin, New Hampshire was repeated in 1967 using comparable methods (Ferris et al., 1971). It was noted that the prevalence of respiratory disease symptoms was lower in 1967 and that, on the average, there was some improvement in pulmonary function. Because there had also been a fall in air pollution between 1961 and 1967, the authors concluded that this was the probable explanation for the observed improvement. In their analysis they were careful to consider other possible explanations for the change, such as observer differences and the increasing use of filter-tip cigarettes.

The second survey in 1967 illustrates the usefulness of repeated prevalence studies in assessing time trends in disease or other population characteristics, provided that comparable measurement methods are used. The effort and expense of keeping a population under continuous long-term surveillance can often be avoided by conducting careful cross-sectional studies at fairly wide intervals.

Example 2: Cardiovascular Disease in Evans County, Georgia

In Chaps. 4 and 5, emphasis has been placed on descriptive epidemiologic findings as a source of hypotheses for further analytic studies. Another very important source of ideas and hypotheses has been clinical observations by astute and concerned health-care professionals. A physician's observations and interest proved to be a major stimulus for the epidemiologic study of cardiovascular disease in Evans County, Georgia, which began in 1960 as a prevalence study (Hames, 1971, Cassel, 1971a and b, McDonough et al., 1965).

Dr. Curtis Hames, who practiced in the area, was impressed with the difference in frequency with which he found coronary heart disease occurring in whites and blacks. Although coronary heart disease was a common problem in his white patients, he rarely saw it in blacks, despite the fact that many black patients had hypertension and appeared to consume a high animal-fat diet. Furthermore, the male-female difference in susceptibility to coronary heart disease which was so obvious in whites was not apparent in blacks.

In order to confirm and explain these differences in a systematic fashion, Hames encouraged the interest and participation of epidemiologists and other investigators. Largely due to his excellent rapport with the community, there was nearly complete participation of the selected study subjects.

Evans County is located on flat or slightly rolling terrain about 60 miles inland from the coastal port of Savannah, Georgia; its greatest diameter is 19 miles. The county's economy was, in 1960, primarily agricultural, although its extensive pine forests were a source of lumber, pulpwood, and turpentine. In 1960, the total population was 6,952, of which 66.5% were white and 33.5% were black.

The study sample consisted of a 50 percent random selection of county residents, aged 15 through 39, and all residents aged 40 and over. Of the 3,377 persons chosen, 92 percent underwent the study examination, which consisted of a medical and dietary history, physical examination, urinalysis, serum-cholesterol measurement, electrocardiogram, and chest x-ray. The social class standing of each subject was determined according to the occupation, education, and source of income of the head of the household.

The diagnosis of coronary heart disease required that a subject have either a history of angina pectoris, a history of myocardial infarction, or electrocardiographic evidence of myocardial infarction. Each of these manifestations was defined as definite, probable, possible, or absent according to standard criteria. It is essential for investigators to establish, adhere to, and describe in study reports, strict criteria for the diagnosis of disease so that others may know just what kinds of cases were included or excluded. Strict criteria also permit other investigators to reproduce the study findings, or at least to understand why their own study results might differ.

The major findings of the Evans County prevalence study included confirmation of the initial clinical observations. Coronary heart disease prevalence was indeed lower in blacks than in whites, the difference occurring only in men. Part of this black-white difference could be explained by social class, since white men of lower socioeconomic status had coronary heart disease prevalence rates approaching the low levels in blacks, almost all of whom were in the lower social bracket. The age-adjusted prevalence rates were:

97 per thousand in high-social-class whites
40 per thousand in low-social-class whites
21 per thousand in blacks

The investigators could not explain these racial and social class differences by taking into account differences in other risk factors, including blood pressure, serum-cholesterol levels, body weight, cigarette smoking, and dietary intake. However, it was noted that habitual physical activity, as estimated by type of occupation, was inversely related to coronary heart disease prevalence. Men in occupations involving the most physical exertion (e.g., manual labor, sharecropping) showed the lowest prevalence of coronary heart disease. Since these occupations were primarily engaged in by blacks and low-social-class whites, it appeared that physical activity might explain their relatively low prevalence of coronary heart disease.

As with the Berlin, New Hampshire study, described above, a second examination procedure was carried out several years later, beginning in 1967. However, this was *not* for the purpose of repeating the prevalence study. Rather, the second round of examinations was applied only to the initially examined cohort as part of the follow-up for an incidence study. An initial prevalence survey can be, and often is, used as the first stage of an incidence study, in that it defines and characterizes a *population at risk*—those initially free of the disease being studied. As will be described in Chap. 8, this population at risk can then be followed up for the development of the disease.

The incidence study confirmed the black-white difference in the occurrence of coronary heart disease, but the social class difference in whites was no longer evident. It appeared that this was due to a rapid catching up of the lower-class men to the upper-class men in coronary heart disease risk, during a period when Evans County was changing from an agrarian to an industrial economy. The only subgroup of white men with the same low risk as the blacks were sharecroppers, again suggesting a protective effect of high levels of physical activity.

REFERENCES

Arkin, H., and R. R. Colton, *Tables for Statisticians, 2d ed.* (New York: Barnes and Noble, 1963), pp. 26–27, 158–161.

Cassel, J. C. 1971a. Summary of major findings of the Evans County cardiovascular studies. *Arch. Intern. Med.*, **128**:887–889.

Cassel, J. C.: 1971b. Review of the 1960 through 1962 cardiovascular disease prevalence study. *Arch. Intern. Med.*, **128**:890–895.

Ferris, B. G., Jr., and D. O. Anderson. 1962. The prevalence of chronic respiratory disease in a New Hampshire town. *Am. Rev. Resp. Dis.*, **86**:165–177.

Ferris, B. G., Jr., I. T. T. Higgins, M. W. Higgins, J. M. Peters, W. F. van Ganse, and M. D. Goldman. 1971. Chronic nonspecific respiratory disease, Berlin, New Hampshire, 1961–1967: a cross-sectional study. *Am. Rev. Resp. Dis.*, **104**:232–244.

Hames, C. G. 1971. Evans County cardiovascular and cerebrovascular epidemiologic study: Introduction. *Arch. Intern. Med.*, **128**:883–886.

Hansen, M. H., W. N. Hurwitz, and W. G. Madow, *Sampling Survey Methods and Theory.* vol. I., Methods and Application. (New York:Wiley 1953), Chaps. 1–3.

Hill, A. B., *Principles of Medical Statistics.* (London: Oxford University Press, 1971), Chaps. 2, 3.

McDonough, J. R., C. G. Hames, S. C. Stulb, and G. E. Garrison. 1965. Coronary heart disease among Negroes and whites in Evans County, Georgia. *J. Chron. Dis.*, **18**:443–468.

Reid, D. D., D. O. Anderson, B. G. Ferris, Jr., and C. M. Fletcher. 1964. An Anglo-American comparison of the prevalence of bronchitis. *Brit. Med. J.*, **2**:1487–1491.

Chapter 7

Case-Control Studies

Case-control studies are closely related to prevalence or cross-sectional studies (discussed in Chap. 6). However, because they generally involve fewer and more readily accessible subjects, case-control studies are much more often carried out. Among analytic studies, they are usually the first approach to determining whether a particular personal characteristic or environmental factor is related to disease occurrence.

How Case-Control Studies Are Carried Out

Identification and Collection of Cases Once the study objectives and methods have been clearly defined, the first step in a case-control study is the identification of the cases or diseased persons to be studied. (Many rightfully object to the use of the term "case" to refer to a sick human being. Although this dehumanizing term should be avoided in the clinical setting, its use facilitates clear communication about research. In this context it does not imply any lack of sympathy or concern about the ill.)

As mentioned previously in connection with prevalence studies, it is important to set up criteria for the diagnosis and inclusion of cases in the investigation and to describe these criteria carefully when the study is finally reported. It is usually advisable to require objective evidence and documentation of the disease, even if, as a result, some cases will have to be omitted and the size of the case group reduced. Thus, for a study of renal calculi, it may be best to insist that all included cases have stones documented by x-ray evidence or removal by surgery, not diagnosed only by the presence of renal colic. By accepting less well-documented cases, the investigator runs the risk of diluting his case group with some noncases and lessening his chances of finding differences between the case group and the control group.

This recommendation, of course, applies to disease identification for all types of studies, not just case-control studies. However, as was stressed in the last section of Chap. 3, *misclassification* of a few nondiseased persons as cases and of a few diseased persons as controls, no matter how distressing to the clinician, will probably not prevent the discovery of major case-control differences.

The cases may be identified or "ascertained" by a community-wide search, but more often, they are limited to those found in one, or perhaps a few, hospitals, clinics, or medical centers. The case group will usually be limited to those seen or diagnosed during a particular time period. For example, one may decide to study all cases of well-documented renal stones seen at a particular hospital during the 2-year period, January 1, 1974 through December 31, 1975.

Usually, it will not be possible to include in the study all the patients who meet the diagnostic criteria and the time and place specifications. There will be a variety of reasons for this. Some patients will have moved away, died, or will refuse to cooperate; or, some hospital records may be lost so that certain essential information is not available to the investigator. He or she, in turn, should report how many cases met the initial criteria for inclusion and how many were finally included. The reasons why some cases had to be omitted and the number of cases omitted for each reason should be stated.

Selection of Control Subjects   The decision as to who will constitute the control group or groups is perhaps the most difficult one to be made in planning a case-control study, and it requires a good deal of skill and judgment. In a prevalence study this problem does not arise since the cases may be compared with the entire nonaffected portion of the population. By settling for the simple low-cost case-control study instead of the large community-wide prevalence study, the investigator gives up the chance of comparing all the diseased and nondiseased persons in the community. However this is done in the hope that almost as much can be learned about the relationship of the disease to other variables by studying a group of cases and a group of controls. Sometimes a relatively small sample derived randomly from the entire population can be utilized as a control group. However obtaining the desired participation of this kind of representative control group is difficult and often not feasible.

General Principles   One of the most important considerations in selecting controls involves the information to be collected concerning study variables or potential etiologic factors. There should be no major differences between case and control groups as to the quality or availability of this information. Availability of information implies both (1) how much information is obtained concerning each case and control, and (2) what proportions of the case and control groups will, or can, supply it. Equal access to important information previously recorded in a similar fashion for both cases and controls—for example, birth weight recorded in the same hospital—may strongly favor the use of a particular control group. If data have to be obtained by interview, then one worries that quality or availability of information may differ due to differences between cases and controls in emotional state, knowledge of the disease studied, educational or socioeconomic status, and location of the interview (e.g., at home or in a hospital).

Consideration of the *known* sources of bias in quality and quantity of information about cases and controls and of the fact that there are often biases which are *unknown* usually leads the investigator to attempt to find controls that are similar in a general way to the cases, except for the essential difference in whether the disease under investigation is present or absent. Yet, this striving for general similarity should not be carried to the point where there is little or no hope of finding case-control differences in the factors under study. For example, by selecting the controls so that they are of similar educational background to the cases, one will minimize case-control differences in the understanding of a written questionnaire. But this selection procedure will also preclude the study of the relation of educational level to the disease and may seriously impair case-control comparisons of factors related to education, such as socioeconomic status.

In selecting a control group two major questions must be answered

1 From what source(s) will controls be drawn?
2 What will be the method of selection of controls from each of these sources?

These decisions must take into account the need, mentioned above, for controls that are generally similar, but not too similar, to the cases, plus some very practical considerations—in particular, the control groups that are potentially available, and the human and financial resources that can be used for the study.

Selecting a Source of Controls   Many sources of controls have been used, including:

1 Patients within the same medical-care facility
   a Without regard to their diagnosis
   b Excluding those with certain diseases
   c Including only those with certain diseases such as mild or "act-of-God" conditions (e.g., hernias, accidental injuries)
   d Examined and found to be healthy
2 Persons drawn from outside the facility
   a Sample of general community
   b Friends or acquaintances
   c Fellow employees
   d Neighbors
   e Family members such as spouses or siblings

When one is faced with the practical decision as to which source of controls to use, reasons for and against any potential source can usually be mustered, and the reasons why the source chosen might have given biased results will be heard from critics after the study is reported. For example, the investigator may decide to select controls for hospitalized renal calculus cases from herniorrhaphy cases in the same hospital, since that hospital serves a particular socioeconomic and ethnic segment of the community, and since, after the acute pain has subsided, the mental status of a kidney stone patient should not be very different from that of a hernia patient (as contrasted with a patient, say, with a stroke or terminal cancer). Yet if an important difference between kidney stone patients and their hernia controls is found, there will usually be the lingering question of whether the difference is related to kidney stones or to hernias. Therefore, it is frequently helpful to have a diagnostically heterogeneous control group, or more than one control group, if possible. Similarly, repetition of the study by other investigators in other settings will usually reveal whether or not some underlying truth about renal calculi has been discovered. MacMahon and Pugh (1970) have thoroughly discussed many of these important issues and other factors to be considered in selecting controls.

Selecting Control Subjects from the Source   Selection of the control group from the chosen source usually involves sampling. If resources are limited, the control group will usually be equal in size to the case group or smaller than the case group, if necessary. If resources permit the inclusion of more study subjects and no more cases are available, the control group may be enlarged to decrease sampling variation by having, for example, twice or three times as many controls as cases, or even more.

As already noted, selecting a source places some general limitations on the nature of the control group. In addition, when individual controls are chosen from the source, the investigator will often *match* the controls to the cases with regard to some important characteristics such as age or sex. By matching on a particular characteristic, the investigator immediately eliminates a case-control difference in this characteristic as a possible contributor to a case-control difference in a study variable. For example, if the cases and controls are matched for age and it is subsequently found that they differ in blood pressure, age could not be the explanation for this blood pressure difference. In the unusual instance that nothing is known about the disease, not even, say, its age and sex distribution, then no matching would be desired since matching precludes any case-control comparison of the matched variable.

Controls are usually picked individually, in a "paired" fashion. That is, for each case, one or more controls is picked in some systematic fashion according to preset rules or criteria. In a study of renal calculi, it may be decided to include as controls other urological patients who have no urinary-tract stones or obvious mental impairment due to uremia or other cause and who are matched to the cases with regard to age, sex, race, and date of admission. The paired selection of a matched control for each case might involve selecting the first patient admitted to the urological service after the case, who meets the diagnostic and mental status criteria, who is of the same sex and race as the case, and whose age differs by no more than 5 years from that of the case. Some leeway is necessary in matching for quantitative variables such as age and admission date, or else no match will be found for most cases. Failure to find matched controls will also occur frequently if matching is attempted on more than a few characteristics.

If the disease being studied is known to be uncommon in the group serving as a source for controls, then little, if any, diagnostic effort or documentation is needed to rule out the disease in the selected controls. However, if the disease could occur commonly in controls, at least some attempt to rule it out, such as an interview question or a quick review of the medical chart, is desirable to minimize misclassification.

Data Collection Any source of data about the study variables may be used. As has been mentioned, accurate information collected on both cases and controls before the disease developed is ideal. Collecting information after the disease develops may be necessary, but every effort should be made to avoid qualitative and quantitative case-control differences in the data gathered. For example, if possible, the research assistant(s) recording laboratory data for all study subjects should do so without knowing whether particular individuals are cases or controls. Similarly it may often be desirable to structure data-collecting interviews to avoid discussing disease status altogether, or at least until the questions about etiologic variables have been asked.

Data Analysis   Normally, the basic case-control comparison is expressed in terms of the proportion of cases versus the proportion of controls who show a particular characteristic. If the characteristic is quantitative rather than a qualitative "yes-or-no" attribute, then its distribution in cases and controls can be compared, as can the more general descriptions of the distribution, such as the mean, standard deviation, and the median.

Interpretation

If the cases show a higher proportion with an attribute than do the controls or if the distributions or mean levels of an attribute differ, then there is an observed association between the attribute and the disease. Interpreting whether this association implies a cause-and-effect relationship is another matter, involving a number of considerations to be discussed in Chap. 11.

It may seem more convenient or natural to think about the study results expressed, as is usually done in a prevalence or incidence study, as the rate of disease occurrence in persons with a particular attribute compared to the disease rate in those either without that attribute or with a different attribute. In case-control studies the results of comparisons are usually expressed in the converse manner, that is, as the relative frequency of the attribute in the diseased versus the nondiseased. Fortunately, the results of case-control studies can be converted mathematically to comparisons of disease rates, or at least to an expression of relative risk of disease, under certain conditions. These are, that cases and controls are reasonably representative of persons with and without disease in the underlying population and that the disease prevalence rate of the underlying population is known, or at least known to be small. The interested reader should refer to MacMahon and Pugh (1970) for a description of these methods.

As with prevalence studies, case-control studies usually involve *existing* disease cases which, as discussed in Chap. 6, p. 80, may differ in a variety of ways from all cases that develop. One way to try to overcome this problem is to include only those cases that first develop or are first diagnosed during the period of data collection. By using only new cases and selecting controls to be representative of the population at risk for developing the disease, the case-control study then aims more directly at determining factors responsible for disease *development*, much like an incidence study. Paradoxically, although this should provide a broader and more representative *spectrum* of cases, it may limit the *number* of cases available for study, resulting in a sample size that is too small to provide reliable data.

It should also be emphasized that the source of cases for the study may be more apt to provide medical care to one type of case than another. For example, cases derived only from a hospital and not from outpatient clinics as well, may have the most severe disease. Thus, while we have emphasized the problems and vagaries of control groups, the characteristics of the case group must also be carefully considered in study design and interpretation.

Example 1: Oral Contraceptives and Thromboembolic Disease

Millions of women now take oral contraceptive tablets to prevent pregnancy. Several questions concerning the safety of these agents have arisen. One of the major areas of concern has been whether or not oral contraceptives predispose to thromboembolic conditions, particularly thrombophlebitis and its possibly fatal sequela, pulmonary embolism. Following the publication of some clinical case reports in the early 1960's it became apparent that epidemiologic studies were necessary to determine whether women who take oral contraceptives are indeed at greater risk of developing these diseases.

Thrombophlebitis and pulmonary embolism *not* secondary to trauma, surgery, or childbirth, develop rather rarely in women during the reproductive years. Thus a prevalence or incidence study of this question seemed impractical, at least as a first approach, since many thousands of women would have to have been studied in order to find an adequate sample of cases. Case-control investigations were therefore undertaken, both in Great Britain and the United States. The U.S. study by Sartwell and his associates is an excellent example of the case-control method.

The investigators decided to include as cases, women, ages 15–44, hospitalized with thromboembolic conditions and discharged alive within the previous 3 years. It was necessary to collect the cases from a large number of hospitals to obtain an adequate sample size. All told, there were 48 participating hospitals in five large eastern cities: Baltimore, New York City, Philadelphia, Pittsburgh, and Washington, D.C. Cases were excluded from the study if they also had a chronic condition possibly predisposing to thromboembolism, such as diabetes mellitus or hypertension, or a recent precipitating event such as surgery, pregnancy, trauma, localized infection, or prolonged inactivity. Reasonable medical evidence for thromboembolism was required, and all cases were reviewed independently by two physicians.

The derivation of the final study group of 175 cases was carefully described by the authors and clearly shows the marked attrition that often occurs between *potential* and *actual* numbers of study subjects. In all, 2,648 women in the desired age range with thromboembolic conditions within 3 years were identified and their hospital records were abstracted. The vast majority of these cases, 2,288, were immediately rejected because of having possibly predisposing conditions, and another 99 were rejected for other reasons, such as sterility (which obviates contraceptive use), death, or having moved from the area. Of the 261 women selected as suitable cases, 72 had to be dropped because the interview could not be obtained and another 14 were excluded because no interview could be obtained from their matched control subjects.

Two matched controls were selected for each case with the expectation that if one could not be interviewed the alternate control would still be available, thus yielding data on one control per case. Matching was done on several criteria:

Hospital	:	same as case
Sex	:	all women
Discharge date	:	same 6-month interval as that of case

Discharge status	:	all alive
Age	:	same 5-year span
Marital status	:	same
Residence	:	(not stated but presumably the same metropolitan area)
Race	:	same
Parity	:	same general class, i.e., no pregnancies, one or two pregnancies, three or more pregnancies
Hospital pay status	:	ward, semiprivate, or private room

Also, controls were excluded in the same manner as the cases, i.e., for chronic diseases possibly predisposing to thromboembolism or for sterility. Most control subjects turned out to have acute medical and surgical illnesses, conditions treated by elective surgery, or traumatic injuries.

Cases and controls were interviewed at home. A variety of questions were asked so as to provide data concerning pertinent variables such as religion, educational level, and smoking habits. To elicit information about contraceptive usage, cases and controls were asked to select from a list of thirteen methods those which they had used within the 2 years before they were hospitalized.

Data analysis showed that the overall frequency of employment of *any* birth-control method was similar in the 175 cases and controls—114 and 101 users of at least one method, respectively—and many women had used more than one method during the 2-year period. While the case-control differences in proportions using each of the other methods were small and not statistically significant, cases did report using oral contraceptives significantly more often than did controls—67 versus 30 women or 38 percent versus 17 percent.

Using a simple formula to compute relative risk, the investigators found that users of oral contraceptives were about four times as likely as nonusers to develop thromboembolic conditions. Furthermore it could be shown that about one-fourth of the total cases would be attributable to oral contraceptive usage if a cause-and-effect relationship were involved. It was, of course, carefully pointed out that the cases studied were a highly selected group, that is, free of predisposing conditions, unlike most thromboembolism cases.

Further analysis showed that the case-control differences in oral-contraceptive use were present in the major subgroups of the study subjects, when the total group was subdivided by such variables as age and marital status. The case-control differences were found for several different thromboembolic conditions including deep thrombophlebitis of the lower extremity, pulmonary embolism, and intracranial vascular conditions.

Example 2: Pedestrians Fatally Injured by Motor Vehicles

In their concern with learning about the diseases which present complex diagnostic or pathophysiologic problems, medical personnel are apt to forget that injuries and death due to gross physical trauma are one of the chief health problems in affluent industrialized societies as well as in "less developed" areas. In particular, accidents are the leading cause of death in children and young adults in the United States. Automobile accidents lead all other types as a cause of death.

The word "accident" implies that physical injuries produced by automobiles and other energy sources are haphazard and uncontrollable. Among those arguing against this fatalistic concept, Haddon has advocated the use of carefully designed and implemented epidemiologic studies as a means of identifying factors responsible for traumatic injuries, so that appropriate preventive measures can be instituted. His research group's interesting study of the characteristics of pedestrians fatally injured by motor vehicles in New York City is an example of the imaginative use of the case-control method to attack a serious and poorly understood problem (Haddon et al., 1961).

At the time of the study in 1959, little was known about pedestrian-associated or "host" factors related to being struck and killed by a car. Substantial funds were being expended for public education programs and other means of "pedestrian control," without much evidence that these were effective preventive measures. The previous findings that many fatally injured pedestrians had been drinking heavily had not been evaluated in comparison to the alcohol consumption of the population at risk or, more simply, to that of noninjured pedestrians. Likewise, the age distribution of killed pedestrians, with relatively high percentages of young children and elderly adults, had not been compared with the age distribution of all or of nonkilled pedestrians, to determine whether the *mortality rate*, or risk of being killed, is actually greater in very young and very old pedestrians. Thus, age and blood-alcohol concentration were included among several characteristics that were measured in fatally injured pedestrians and their matched controls in the study to be described.

New York City was a very appropriate place for this investigation. Pedestrian deaths were relatively frequent, and they accounted for about 70 percent of all fatalities in motor vehicle accidents. The case series consisted of 50 adults (18 years of age and older) who were struck and killed by automobiles in Manhattan between May 3, 1959 and November 7, 1959. Autopsy confirmation of the cause of death was required. Of 57 cases initially considered, the 7 omissions consisted of 2 who were killed by bicycles, 1 who was purposely pushed into the path of a car, 1 with unknown site or time of the accident, 1 who died of a coronary occlusion while convalescing from the accident, and 2 who were omitted because of clerical errors.

Four matched controls were selected for each case by visiting each accident site at a later date, but on the same day of the week and as close as possible to the time of day when the accident occurred. All but eight site visits for control selection were completed within 6 weeks of the accident. Thus, controls were matched to the cases for accident site and time. In addition, controls were matched to the accident cases for sex and were limited, as were the cases, to adults.

The practical problems involved in this form of "shoe-leather" epidemiology can best be communicated by the investigators' own description of the control selection and interview procedures

> The site visits were made by a team of two or three of the authors and one to four medical students working at each location with one or two uniformed members of the Police Department Accident Investigation Squad (A.I.S.).

In visiting each site one of three basic approaches was used. In the first type, that used in many busy neighborhoods, for example, opposite Grand Central Station on a weekday at 6:10 P.M., the entire team arrived and immediately stopped the *first* 4 adult pedestrians of the same sex as the deceased. At such busy sites the group arrived and accomplished its purposes in 5 minutes or less from start to finish.

When the accident site was in a neighborhood in which it was suspected that the group might be seen and avoided, a second approach was used. Under such circumstances, for example, at sites in the Bowery, the group arrived and 'swept the block' stopping successively the *first* 4 adult pedestrians of the required sex who were headed toward or away from the accident site. By pedestrian here and throughout this report is meant a person progressing by walking, not lounging stationary, sitting, or lying down.

In the third approach, used where pedestrian traffic was very light, for example at 108th Street and the East River (F.D.R.) Drive at 1:40 A.M., the group would lounge nearby or sit in a car at or near the site watching for approaching pedestrians, and as each of the *first* 4 of these came into view he, or, where appropriate, she, was quickly approached and stopped.

The site visited was the sidewalk point closest to the exact location of the accident as described on the police or medical examiner's report. For example, one report indicated that the deceased had been crossing the street 40 feet from a given corner. This was found to be directly in front of a 'rathskeller', and it was at that point that the first 4 pedestrians were stopped.

Great care was taken to avoid any attempt at matching for the characteristics of the deceased, except in so far as sex and adulthood were concerned. In addition, for methodologic uniformity, at all sites the same investigator pointed out to the accompanying police each individual to be stopped. Although the exact details varied with the circumstances, the person was immediately approached and told by the policeman, 'Please step over for a minute while the doctors ask you a few questions.' A nearby member of the team immediately stepped up and began talking uninterruptedly: 'I don't want to know your name; I merely want to ask you a few questions. Do you live in Manhattan?' The interview was usually easily begun in this manner, although 12 refusals occurred (for each of which the next pedestrian was substituted) . . . .

This investigation was carried out without publicity of any kind. With one exception it was invariably possible to stop the members of each pedestrian sample prior to the formation of the substantial group of watchers which sometimes formed thereafter. The exception, in a 'tough' neighborhood at 2:30 A.M., involved the only site at which 2 persons had been fatally injured in the same accident. On arrival, it was possible to obtain quickly the first 7 but not the eighth interview and specimen of breath, a small, hostile crowd quickly forming from an adjacent bar. As a result, only the first 4 of the 7 interviews and specimens obtained at this site were used, being counted twice in the analyses of the data.

The interview included questions as to: place and length of residence; place of birth; age; present occupation; and marital status. Sex, apparent race, appearance and apparent sobriety, date, location, time of interview, and weather were also recorded.

Immediately on finishing the interview the interviewer stated approximately as follows, 'I only have one more thing for you to do (and then you can go) and that is to blow up this bag for me.' Simultaneously he removed a Saran bag from an envelope and showed the pedestrian how to place one of its two ends in his mouth and blow until told to stop. This finished, the pedestrian was thanked and told that the interview was over.

A large percentage of those interviewed were foreign born, and many of these admitted to no knowledge of English. Rather than weaken the investigation by omitting these pedestrians when no member of the team knew a common language, passersby were stopped and asked to serve as interpreters. Apparently because those walking in the same neighborhoods or, in some cases, accompanying those stopped (many of the latter being interviewed themselves) tended to know the same languages, this procedure proved very satisfactory. With its use no one failed to be interviewed because of a language barrier and interviews were completed in Armenian, German, Greek, Spanish, and other languages and dialects.

As implied above, blood-alcohol concentrations were measured by analysis of breath specimens and the other data concerning the controls were recorded as described. Data concerning the cases were obtained chiefly from official records describing the accidents.

Postmortem blood-alcohol measurements were studied in those cases who survived less than 6 hours after the accident.

Data analysis for the case-control comparison revealed that, indeed, fatally injured pedestrians were older than the controls, their mean ages being 58.8 years and 41.6 years, respectively. Additional data collected later showed nonfatally injured pedestrians to be intermediate in age, with a mean of 48.4 years. Thus, advancing age appeared to increase the pedestrian's risk both of being struck by a car and of dying once struck.

Regarding the effects of alcohol, significantly higher blood-alcohol concentrations were found in cases than controls. Appreciable increases in risk were noted even at the relatively low levels of 10 to 40 mg/100 cc. Putting together the age and alcohol data it appeared that there were two relatively discrete high-risk groups—the elderly who had been drinking little if any alcohol and the middle-aged who had been drinking heavily.

It was also found that the case group was more often foreign-born and of lower socioeconomic status than the controls, and less often married. However these differences could be explained by age differences between the case and control groups. Weather conditions, rain in particular, did not appear to be associated to any substantial degree with traffic deaths.

In addition to the case-control comparisons, information about the fatally injured group itself was of interest and importance. Only a small percentage lived outside of Manhattan and were commuters or out-of-town visitors. While the accidents were scattered about the city, most occurred outside of major business and shopping areas. The accidents occurred most frequently in the evening and night hours, suggesting the importance of emergency medical care during this time of day.

Evaluation and Role of the Case-Control Method

Case-control studies are the most readily and cheaply carried out of all analytic epidemiologic studies. For rare diseases they may be the only practical approach. Yet the problems involved in selecting appropriate control groups and collecting comparable information on cases and controls are often of such magnitude that the results of case-control studies are open to a variety of legitimate questions and objections, generally more so than the results of prevalence and incidence studies.

Case-control studies have played a vital role in the development of many fruitful lines of study. For example the relationship of cigarette smoking to lung cancer was demonstrated in case-control studies before any incidence studies of this question were carried out. Because of their low cost, case-control studies should often be the first approach to the testing of a hypothesis. Similarly, they are useful for an exploratory study of a variety of variables (sometimes referred to as a "fishing expedition") to find clues and leads for further study.

REFERENCES

Haddon, W., Jr., P. Valien, J. R. McCarroll, and C. J. Umberger. 1961. A controlled investigation of the characteristics of adult pedestrians fatally injured by motor vehicles in Manhattan. *J. Chron. Dis.*, **14**:655–678.

MacMahon, B., and T. F. Pugh, *Epidemiology: Principles and Methods.* (Boston: Little, Brown, 1970), Chap. 12.

Sartwell, P. E., A. T. Masi, F. G. Arthes, G. R. Greene, and H. E. Smith. 1969. Thromboembolism and oral contraceptives: An epidemiologic case-control study. *Am. J. Epidemiology*, **90**:365–380.

Chapter 8

Incidence or Cohort Studies

Of the various types of observational epidemiologic studies, *incidence* or *cohort* studies are generally thought to provide the most definitive information about disease etiology. They do provide the most direct measurement of the *risk of disease development.* However, if carried out prospectively, they can be expensive and time-consuming, requiring a long-term commitment of funds and dedicated personnel. Furthermore, as will be discussed, they are not free of potential biases and other scientific problems.

How Incidence Studies Are Carried Out

Defining the Study Population Initially, a study population or cohort is identified. This population is to be followed up over a period of time for the development of the disease(s) under investigation. The cohort chosen may be a rather general population group, such as the residents of a community, or a more specialized population that can readily be studied such as an occupational group or group of insured persons. Or, the cohort may be selected because of a known exposure to a suspected etiologic factor such as a source of ionizing radiation or a drug or pesticide. If exposure to the suspected factor characterizes all or virtually all cohort members, then a similar but unexposed cohort or some other standard of comparison is required to evaluate the experience of the exposed group.

The incidence study focuses on disease development. In order for a disease to develop, it must, of course, be absent initially. Thus the study population must be shown, in some way, to be free of the disease, that is, to be a population at risk for disease development. For a rare, rapidly fatal disease such as acute leukemia, a few cases initially present in the population will probably be self-evident. For a more common disease such as coronary heart disease in middle-aged men, an initial examination of the potential study population may be required to find and exclude existing cases of disease. As illustrated by the Evans County study (Chap. 6), this initial examination may be part of a prevalence study.

An initial examination may serve another important purpose. In it, some or all of the potential etiologic factors and other pertinent study variables may be measured. Nevertheless, some cohort studies with certain specific objectives do not require an initial examination since the data necessary to characterize the study subjects are available from other sources.

Follow-up　Once the population is initially defined and the appropriate characteristics of its members have been assessed, the population must be followed up for the development of the disease. Follow-up procedures vary from study to study both in intensity and completeness, depending on the disease manifestations to be measured.

Simple, relatively complete follow-up is available for life-insurance-company investigations of factors affecting mortality. For their purposes, death is the only end-point of importance, and it must be reported to the company in order for the policy benefits to be paid.

On the other hand, follow-up to detect all new cases of coronary heart disease or stroke may require several different procedures, including periodic reexaminations, surveillance of deaths, hospitalizations, and physicians' office visits, and correspondence with subjects who have moved from the area. However, limitations on available resources may dictate that only a portion of all possible follow-up procedures be used, perhaps just hospitalizations and deaths, for example. Even though incomplete, such partial follow-up may be perfectly adequate for the purposes of the study.

The duration of follow-up required is determined primarily by the number of disease cases needed to provide reliable, statistically significant answers to the specific questions under study. This can usually be determined in advance, once the study population size and the disease incidence rate is known. For example, if the study population contains 1,000 persons and the incidence rate is 1 percent per year, about 10 new cases may be expected during each year of follow-up. If 100 cases are needed to provide answers with a certain degree of reliability, then the study may be expected to last about 10 years.

This example is somewhat oversimplified and does not take into account such factors as a possible reduction over the years in the number of new cases per year, due to losses of subjects to follow-up, or a possible increase in new cases per year as the population ages, if the incidence increases with age. Although it is often most practical to keep follow-up as short as possible, a study may be designed specifically with a long follow-up period in mind to assess factors which cause or predict disease in the distant future.

During the follow-up period it may be possible to repeat the initial measurements of population characteristics. In this way disease development may be studied in relation both to initial characteristics and to *changes* in these characteristics. For example, it is not only of interest to know whether serum cholesterol level is related to subsequent coronary heart disease, but also whether a *rising* level or a *falling* level adds additional predictive information.

There are other reasons for reassessing population characteristics in the follow-up period. During a long-term study there may be technological improvements in the measuring devices that were used initially. Also, new scientific information about the disease may indicate the importance of measuring additional variables that were not included at first.

Data Analysis As in a prevalence study, the population is subdivided or classified according to the variables that are to be related to the disease. The disease incidence rate is determined for each subgroup, and the rates are compared to see whether the presence or absence (or differences in level, if quantitative) of the variable is related to subsequent disease development. If the study population is a special cohort exposed to a suspected etiologic factor, then its disease incidence is compared to that in a similar nonexposed cohort or to that in the general population.

If all or virtually all study population members are followed up for the same period of time, then a simple overall incidence rate can be used. For example, if the period is uniformly 3 years, then the 3-year incidence rate may be computed for each subgroup. If there are substantial differences among study subjects in length of follow-up, these will have to be taken into account in the data analysis. Follow-up durations may differ markedly when subjects are lost to follow-up before the study is complete—if, for example, they move out of the area or die. Also, some investigations require that new subjects be added to the study population over a relatively long period of time. As a result, if disease incidence is determined up to a specific point in time, subjects will have been followed up for different durations from their time of entry into the study.

The standard method of handling variable follow-up periods involves the use of "person-years" of observation in the denominator of the incidence rate (or person-months or person-days, etc., if more appropriate or convenient). With this approach, each subject contributes only as many years of observation to the population at risk as he is actually observed; if he leaves after 1 year, he contributes 1 person-year; if after 10, 10 person-years.

The assumption involved in adding all subjects' person-years into one denominator is that the disease risk remains relatively constant over time. That is, the third year of observation, for example, is not appreciably different as to disease risk from the first; or, stated in another way, following up three persons for 1 year is equivalent to following up one person for 3 years. The validity of this assumption for any particular study should be considered in evaluating the person-years approach.

Another feature of the person-year method is that one person may contribute person years of observation to more than one subgroup. Suppose, for example, that in a 5-year study, disease incidence is determined for age-decade subgroups. A person entering the study population at age 48 will contribute two person-years of observation to the 40–49-year-old subgroup and three person-years of observation to the 50–59-year-old subgroup. This may also happen with other measurements if they change over time. A person may spend a few years in a particular quartile of serum cholesterol and then shift to a higher or lower quartile.

Interpretation and Evaluation of Incidence Studies

The emphasis in incidence studies is on the prediction of disease development. This type of investigation clearly demonstrates the time sequence between the presence or absence of a factor and the subsequent occurrence of the disease. However, even the prediction of disease does not necessarily imply a cause and effect relationship, as will be discussed in Chap. 11. Furthermore, as has been pointed out, factors associated with a disease can be shown to precede and thus predict the disease in prevalence and case-control studies as well.

A problem that has been emphasized with prevalence and case-control studies is the likelihood of overrepresentation of cases of long duration. This will not be a problem with incidence studies having complete and comprehensive follow-up; the full spectrum of the disease should be available for study.

Despite their good reputation, incidence studies can be subject to important biases. We have mentioned how, in a prevalence or case-control study, the presence or absence of disease may affect the factor under investigation or the measurement of that factor, using the example of cancer and its effects on one's emotional state. In a somewhat analogous fashion, the converse problem may be present in an incidence study. That is, the presence or absence of a study factor may affect the subsequent assessment of disease. This may be especially prone to occur if the decision as to the presence or absence of disease is made by persons who are aware of the subject's status with regard to the study factor.

In a stroke study, for example, it is clearly possible for knowledge of a subject's prior blood pressure to influence, consciously or unconsciously, the decision as to whether or not a stroke has occurred. If this happens, the study will have a built-in correlation between blood pressure and stroke incidence. Similarly, if in a study of cancer, disease detection depends partly upon the initiative or cooperation of the subjects in seeking an examination, those with a family history of cancer or those who smoke might be especially motivated to have a checkup. This can result in bias or in a built-in correlation of the disease with a family history of cancer or with smoking. Thus, every effort should be made to ensure that disease development is detected or decided upon independently of the possible etiologic factors under investigation.

Incidence studies are also subject to possible biases due to loss of study subjects. Such losses may occur initially, if a portion of the target study population does not participate, or later on as members of the study population are lost to follow-up. Marked losses of either type do not necessarily invalidate the study. However, the investigators should consider whether the reasons for loss of subjects might reasonably have affected the study outcome. Sometimes it is possible to gather outside information concerning lost subjects, particularly whether they left due to illness or death or for any reason that might be related to the variables and the disease under investigation.

Example 1: The Framingham Study

Considering the barrage of information about "coronary risk factors" to which the public has been subjected, it may come as a surprise to health-care personnel now in training that only a few decades ago, atherosclerosis and its clinical consequences were generally viewed by the medical profession as degenerative changes that were an inevitable consequence of aging. However, by the late 1940's, descriptive epidemiologic findings and clinical observations were beginning to convince public health authorities that environmental factors might be playing an important role in the disease and that, as a result, prevention was a real possibility. Because of the major importance of coronary heart disease as a cause of disability and death in this country, the U.S. Public Health Service decided to undertake a major long-term incidence study to better define the factors producing this disease.

When the Framingham Study began, around 1950, Framingham, Massachusetts was a town of about 28,000 inhabitants. There were several reasons for selecting this location for the study. At the time, it was a relatively self-contained community with both industrial and rural areas. In this and other ways it was not obviously atypical. There were sufficient numbers of residents in the desired age range to provide an adequate study group. There was evidence, both from a successful previous study of tuberculosis in the community, and from discussions with medical and lay residents, that the townspeople would be cooperative. The area of the town was sufficiently small that the residents could come to one central examining facility. Follow-up of hospitalizations would be relatively easy since most occurred at one central hospital in the town. Furthermore, Framingham was only 20 miles from major medical centers in Boston; thus, medical and scientific consultation would be readily available.

The study was planned to last for 20 years, in view of the slow development of atherosclerosis and its consequences. A long "incubation period" is believed to characterize many of the chronic noninfectious diseases and argues for a long-term study to identify predisposing factors early in life.

The lower and upper age limits of the study population were set at 30 and 60 years. It was felt that older persons should be excluded since many of them already had extensive coronary atherosclerosis and, as a result, to study them would reveal only immediate precipitating factors for clinical events. Persons under thirty were excluded primarily because their incidence of coronary heart disease would be very low and they were a more mobile, hard-to-follow group.

In selecting the study sample, the goal was a group of about 5,000, since this size sample in the 30–60-year age range would produce adequate numbers of cases over the 20-year follow-up period. Knowing that there would be some nonresponse, the investigators selected a larger systematic sample comprising two-thirds of the 10,000 residents of the appropriate ages. The list of town residents was arranged according to precinct, and within each precinct by family according to family-size groups (one member, two members, three or more members, ages 30–60). Two out of every three families were selected. Selection of *families* rather than individuals was a wise decision since (1) one member of a family in the study's age range would not be denied an examination service offered to another member of the same family, (2) many reluctant men received examinations because of being "persuaded" by their more cooperative wives to go to the clinic at the same time, and (3) studies of spouse pairs and familial aggregation of characteristics would be fostered.

The 6,507 members of the sample were invited to participate in the study by town residents who recruited subjects living in their own neighborhoods. These recruiters were part of a group of volunteers who were given a cardiovascular examination at the clinic before the study officially began. Having experienced the examination that was to be given in the study, the volunteer recruiters would be able to describe it to the invited subjects on the basis of personal experience.

Despite this personal approach only 4,469, or about two-thirds of the sample, participated. A group of 740 volunteers were added, yielding a total of 5,209 subjects. The initial examination revealed that 82 subjects already had clinically evident coronary heart disease. These were excluded from the population at risk, leaving a total of 5,127.

This study population has been offered a relatively complete examination every 2 years since the study began. The examination has included a medical history, physical examination, and pertinent laboratory tests such as electrocardiogram, chest x-ray, and serum lipid levels. It has been directed primarily at detecting the development of coronary heart disease and other atherosclerotic conditions such as stroke and peripheral vascular disease. Variables to be related to disease development have also been measured every 2 years. As new types of measurements have acquired importance in this area of research, they have been added to the examination. Thus the investigators have not been limited to the first examination as their only source of information about possible etiologic variables.

Every effort has been made to maintain rapport with the community and with the medical profession in the town. Subjects are kept waiting as little as possible during the examination. A complete report of the examination findings has been sent to each subject's personal physician. No medical care or advice is given by the study's examining physicians except that persons with newly discovered serious abnormalities are advised to contact their own physicians.

Although the biennial examinations at the clinic have been the chief source of follow-up information, disease development has been detected by other means as well. These additional sources include records of hospitalizations and of local physicians' office visits, and information about deaths from death certificates, coroner's reports, and reports of relatives. The diagnosis of any disease studied has been made according to strict criteria so as to include only definite cases in the diseased group.

Maintaining a continuing program of biennial examinations for a few thousand persons has involved a major investment in the operation of the study clinic. A staff of physicians, nurses, laboratory technicians, receptionists, clerical personnel, and others have been necessary for the smooth operation of the clinic and to assure the collection of complete and accurate data. Epidemiologically oriented physicians and statisticians located both on-site and at the National Heart and Lung Institute headquarters in Bethesda, Maryland have carried out the research analyses of data and the preparation of scientific papers.

The study findings have emerged in a large series of reports over the years since 1951 and can only be summarized briefly here. Several representative papers are listed in the references under the first authors, Dawber, Kannel, Gordon, and Friedman.

The study has been able to confirm in great detail that the atherosclerotic diseases do not strike persons at random as they age, but that highly susceptible individuals can be identified in advance of any definite clinical manifestations. Indications of susceptibility, or "risk factors," that have been found in the Framingham Study and other epidemiologic investigations include male sex, advancing age, high serum lipid concentrations, high blood pressure, cigarette smoking, diabetes mellitus (or even milder degrees of carbohydrate intolerance), obesity, low vital capacity, and certain electrocardiographic abnormalities. Other risk factors that have been emphasized more by other studies include certain psychosocial factors, family history of coronary heart disease, and physical inactivity.

The detailed information and large population available at Framingham have permitted more intensive investigation of the unique role of each risk factor. For example, it was found that obesity is not related equally to all manifestations of coronary heart disease. Although it does appear to predispose to angina pectoris and to sudden unexpected death, it is not related to myocardial infarction per se. Also, sufficient numbers of cases emerged to permit the study of interrelationships of several risk factors. One important finding was that persons with combinations of risk factors (for example hypertensive male smokers with high serum lipid levels) are at especially high risk of developing coronary heart disease.

As the study population ages, more emphasis can be placed on the diseases of the elderly such as stroke. Furthermore, the wide scope of information collected in Framingham has permitted the epidemiologic study of other nonatherosclerotic diseases as well, for example, rheumatic heart disease, gout, and gallbladder disease. In addition, several studies of epidemiologic methods have been carried out there.

At present the major research efforts in the epidemiology of coronary heart disease are being switched more and more from observational studies, of which Framingham has been one of the most important, to experimental trials attempting actually to lower the risk of disease. The predictive value of serum lipids, blood pressure, and cigarette smoking have been repeatedly demonstrated. Many feel that it is now necessary to prove that actively changing these characteristics by diet, drugs, and other means will safely lower risk and prevent or postpone atherosclerotic disease before widespread measures are applied to the general public or to high-risk individuals. Thus, at the time of this writing the National Institutes of Health is initiating a large-scale Multiple Risk Factor

Intervention Trial which will be a controlled experiment (see Chap. 9) to evaluate active preventive measures, involving the collaboration of several medical centers in the United States.

While it is generally accepted, then, that enough has been learned about factors predisposing to coronary heart disease to justify serious attempts at prevention, this does not mean that observational epidemiologic studies and other efforts to identify causal factors are no longer needed. There are many individuals developing the disease who by present criteria are at low risk. Conversely, many persons in the apparent high risk groups remain free of clinical coronary heart disease. Thus, our power to predict coronary heart disease is limited, and further studies are needed to identify pertinent risk factors.

Example 2: Mortality in Radiologists—Does Radiation Shorten Their Lives?

As the use of man-made sources of ionizing radiation has increased, so has the concern that these may be producing a variety of adverse effects on life and health (MacMahon, 1967; Whittenberger, 1967). While intense acute exposures have clearly proved to be quite harmful or even fatal, the evidence is less obvious regarding the consequences of chronic exposure to relatively low levels of radiation. Experimental animals subjected to chronic exposure have died sooner than expected, but findings in animals are not always applicable to man.

The effects on man's life-span are clearly a matter requiring epidemiologic study. Laboratory investigations of radiation effects on animals, cells, and other biological or biochemical systems, however important and illuminating, do not answer the basic question, *Does exposure to mild and moderate levels of radiation actually shorten human lives?*

Since the intentional exposure of human beings to radiation for the sole purpose of answering this question is ethically unthinkable, one problem for the epidemiologist is to locate human groups who have been or are being exposed for other reasons, so that their mortality experience may be investigated. Groups already studied for a relationship between ionizing radiation and overall mortality or cancers of various types include uranium miners, residents of Hiroshima and Nagasaki who survived the atom bomb, patients receiving radiation therapy for noncancerous conditions such as enlargement of the thymus gland or ankylosing spondylitis, and children exposed in utero to diagnostic x-rays of their mothers' abdomen and pelvis.

Radiologists have also been studied for possible life-shortening effects. Since the findings of some of the earlier studies of radiologists were inconclusive, either because of small numbers of subjects or because of questionable comparison groups and measures of outcome, Seltser and Sartwell (1965) undertook a study of all members of an organization of radiologists compared to members of other medical specialty societies.

The Radiological Society of North America was the radiologists' organization studied. Founded in 1915, it existed during some of the early years of radiology when many radiologists were much less concerned and self-protective about radiation exposure than they have been more recently. (Some of the old-time radiologists even placed their own hand next to the patient routinely, so that its image on the x-ray photograph would help in judging the exposure time.) It was hypothesized in advance that the radiologists were the high-exposure, *high-risk* medical specialty group. The American College of Physicians has been composed largely of internists and was studied as a probable *intermediate-risk* group, since some physicians in this group have fluoroscoped patients to aid in diagnosis. The hypothesized *low-risk* specialty society was the American Academy of Ophthalmology and Otolaryngology, whose membership would contain only a few persons exposed routinely to radiation.

This investigation is described here as an example of a *retrospective* cohort study, contrasting greatly with the Framingham Study in scope and expense. In this study, all the events to be studied had already taken place and the required data were already recorded.

Because the data were already recorded does not mean that preparing them for analysis was an easy task. Several years of work were required to extract the necessary information from the files of the specialty societies and the American Medical Association's Directory Department. All specialists studied were traced from the time of joining their societies in or after 1915 until the end of 1958, and the time and place of death for all deceased members were noted. The cause of death was determined for over 99 percent of the deceased subjects by obtaining death certificates or reviewing other death records. The study was limited to men.

The end point of this study was, of course, mortality. The data were analyzed in terms of person-years of observation. Each physician was considered to have contributed one-half person-year of observation during the year he joined—a convenient approximation which represents the average—plus a full person-year for each subsequent calendar year survived through 1958. Subjects dying before the end of 1958 were credited with one-half year during the year they died, again a convenient approximation. All told, there were 16,339 physician specialists studied, of whom 3,521 were radiologists. Person-years of observation totaled 232,708, of which the radiologists contributed 48,895.

Mortality rates were summarized for three age groups, 35–49 years, 50–64 years, and 65–79 years as well as for the total group. Similarly, mortality experience was looked at in three separate time periods, 1935–1944, 1945–1954, and 1955–1958.

As hypothesized, the death rate was highest among radiologists, intermediate in internists, and lowest in ophthalmologists and otolaryngologists. The differences were larger in the earlier time periods than in later ones and more apparent in older than in younger men. In fact, after 1944, radiologists in the 35–49-year group showed no increase in mortality over the other specialists of the same age.

The authors interpreted these age and time relationships as being consistent with a cumulative harmful effect of x-ray exposure becoming manifest in later life, and a decreasing or disappearing effect in more recent years due to improvements in equipment, techniques, and safety measures.

It was of interest that the radiologists' death rates were similar to those of all U.S. white males. Since physicians are, on the average, of higher socioeconomic status and probably receive better medical care, they would be expected to show a lower mortality rate than all males. This illustrates the importance of selecting appropriate comparison groups when special cohorts, such as radiologists or other occupational groups, are followed up. Comparison with all men would have revealed no mortality difference. The more appropriate comparison, with other medical specialists, *did* reveal a difference.

Putting the age-specific death rates into one cross-sectional analysis of life expectancy starting at age 40 (see Chap. 5, p. 57) was another way of looking at the data. This revealed a similar relationship to medical specialty. The median age at death for 40-year-olds starting in the three successive time periods, 1935–1944, 1945–1954, and 1955–1958, respectively, were radiologists—71.4, 72.0, and 73.5 years; internists—73.4, 74.8, and 76.0 years; and otolaryngologists and ophthalmologists—76.2, 76.0, and 76.4 years.

Recognizing the limitations of death-certificate diagnoses, the investigators noted that the causes of death for each medical specialist group would probably have been recorded with reasonably equal accuracy. They compared the rates for major causes such as cardiovascular disease and cancer. The mortality ratios for major causes in radiologists as compared to ophthalmologists and otolaryngologists were relatively close to the overall ratio of 1.4 for all deaths.

Leukemia showed a higher mortality ratio—2.5, based on 19 *observed* leukemia deaths in the radiologists as compared to the 7.7 *expected* if the eye and ear group's mortality rates had applied to the radiologists. This is consistent with the results of other studies showing that radiation increases the risk of developing leukemia. It was pointed out, though, that the approximate 11 excess deaths from leukemia (19 observed minus 7.7 expected) constituted only a small fraction of the 228 total excess deaths. Thus, the higher death rate in radiologists appeared to be largely a nonspecific across-the-board increase.

In evaluating the findings, the investigators considered other possible sources of the mortality differences among the specialties, such as place of residence and initial self-selection of a medical specialty on the basis of health. The additional information available suggested that these factors did not account for the relatively shorter life expectancy of radiologists and that occupational exposure to ionizing radiation was the most likely explanation.

The investigators stressed, rightfully, that their findings were enhanced by the fact that they had predicted the outcome in advance. This deserves special emphasis because of the fact that epidemiologists and other scientists can be trapped by the so-called post hoc, or after-the-fact, explanation. Given a set of findings or measurements, the human mind is usually ingenious enough to produce a reasonable theory or explanation as to why they occurred. This is accomplished with special ease in fields like medicine or psychology which deal with systems of great complexity. Quite plausible explanations can be brought forth to explain diametrically opposite observations, and almost any result can be made to appear consistent with someone's pet theory. A much better test of a theory is whether it will predict specific outcomes of a study *in advance.*

This is not meant to detract from the importance of exploring data in order to develop new hypotheses or theories for further study. However, once such hypotheses are arrived at, they sooner or later will have to be tested to see whether they *predict* study outcomes.

Role of Incidence Studies

It should be clear from the description of the Framingham Study why prospective incidence studies of general populations are infrequently carried out. They are difficult and expensive, and require the initial willingness to make a long-term commitment and the continuing patience on the part of both the sponsoring agencies and the study personnel. Yet the investment may well prove its worth in the depth and variety of information that such a study can produce.

The need for either a long-term follow-up or a very large study population or both, rests fundamentally on the fact that most diseases studied in this manner have surprisingly low incidence rates. Coronary heart disease is the leading cause of death in the United States, and coronary atherosclerosis is well known to be common in middle-aged men at autopsy. Yet, the incidence of new *clinically identified* cases of coronary heart disease in middle-aged men is only about 1 percent per year. Similarly, although hypertension is a highly *prevalent* condition in U.S. adults, many hypertensives seem to have drifted gradually into their present state, making it difficult both to define and to find *new* cases in a population for an incidence study.

Retrospective incidence studies, of course, can be accomplished relatively quickly if suitable cohorts can be identified and if adequate data about them are available. Yet many diseases of interest are so rare that case-control studies currently represent the only practical epidemiologic approach to studying them.

It now appears that technological changes will increase the feasibility of cohort studies in the future. Storage of medical and demographic information in computer data banks is becoming an accepted approach to improving the efficiency and quality of medical care. A by-product will be the increased availability of information about a variety of cohorts that can be studied both retrospectively and prospectively. On-going efforts in the area of "record-linkage" (i.e., the combination of a variety of records about each person, such as birth, physical examination, illness, and death records) will increase the number of different relationships that can be studied—relationships between a variety of initial characteristics and a variety of disease outcomes.

REFERENCES

Dawber, T. R., and W. B. Kannel. 1962. Atherosclerosis and you: Pathogenetic implications from epidemiologic observations. *J. Am. Geriat.*, **10**:805–821.

Dawber, T. R., W. B. Kannel, and L. P. Lyell. 1963. An approach to longitudinal studies in a community: The Framingham study. *Ann. N.Y. Acad. Sci.*, **107**:539–556.

Friedman, G. D., W. B. Kannel, and T. R. Dawber. 1966. The epidemiology of gallbladder disease: Observations in the Framingham study. *J. Chron. Dis.*, **19**:273–292.

Friedman, G. D., W. B. Kannel, T. R. Dawber, and P. M. McNamara. 1967. An evaluation of follow-up methods in the Framingham heart study. *Am. J. Public Health*, **57**:1015–1024.

Gordon, T., and W. B. Kannel. 1972. Predisposition to atherosclerosis in the head, heart, and legs. *J. Am. Med. Assoc.*, **221**:661–666.

Kannel, W. B., An epidemiologic study of cerebrovascular disease, in *Cerebral Vascular Diseases, 5th Conference*, edited by C. H. Millikan et al. (New York: Grune and Stratton, 1966), pp. 53–66.

Kannel, W. B., W. P. Castelli, and P. M. McNamara. 1967. The coronary profile: 12-year follow-up in the Framingham study. *J. Occup. Med.*, **9**:611–619.

Kannel, W. B., T. R. Dawber, A. Kagan, N. Revotskie, and J. Stokes. 1961. Factors of risk in the development of coronary heart disease: six-year follow-up experience: The Framingham study. *Ann. Intern. Med.*, **55**:33–50.

Kannel, W. B., E. J. LeBauer, T. R. Dawber, and P. M. McNamara. 1967. Relation of body weight to development of coronary heart disease: The Framingham study. *Circulation*, **35**:734–744.

MacMahon, B., Cancer. Chap. 24 in *Preventive Medicine*, edited by D. W. Clark and B. MacMahon, (Boston: Little, Brown, 1967), pp. 423–426.

Whittenberger, J. L., The physical and chemical environment. Chap. 34 in *Preventive Medicine*, edited by D. W. Clark and B. MacMahon, (Boston: Little, Brown, 1967), pp. 630–638.

Seltser, R., and P. E. Sartwell. 1965. The influence of occupational exposure to radiation on the mortality of American radiologists and other medical specialists. *Am. J. Epidemiology*, **81**:2–22.

Chapter 9

Experimental Studies

Experimental studies resemble incidence studies in that they require follow-up of the subjects to determine outcome. However, the essential distinguishing feature of experiments is that they involve some *action* or *manipulation* or *intervention* on the part of the investigators; that is, something is done to at least some of the study subjects. This contrasts with incidence and other observational studies, where the investigators take no action, but only observe.

Experiments are believed to be the best test of a cause-and-effect relationship. Something is done to an *experimental group* and the observed outcome is presumed to be the effect of that action, provided that the same outcome did not occur in an equivalent *control group* that was not acted upon. A cause-and-effect relationship can also be demonstrated by *removing* or *reducing* the alleged causal factor in the experimental group and showing a disappearance or reduction in the effect, while no change is observed in the control group.

The latter approach is especially relevant to epidemiologic experiments in preventive medicine (Hutchison, 1967). If a factor is removed or reduced and the disease incidence declines as a result, the factor is, for practical purposes, a causal one.

Although great value is placed on experimental evidence, experimental studies are often exceedingly difficult to carry out. In addition, they raise some ethical issues which must be considered.

Ethical Problems

In observational studies, the investigator's chief ethical problem, aside from the need for objectivity and conscientious work, is to maintain the confidentiality of his records about each person studied. Harm might come to an individual if some of his characteristics, recorded in confidence for medical or scientific purposes, were made available to others, or were communicated to the individual, himself, in an inappropriate manner. In the main, though, the observational epidemiologist is a passive observer of nature with few ethical problems.

The experimentalist's ethical position is quite different, since he takes it upon himself to do something to people. He must have good reason to believe that what he proposes to do has an excellent chance of helping them. On the other hand, he must also have ample doubt about the value of what is to be done, compared to doing nothing or doing what had been done in the past. Otherwise he could not, in good conscience, subject the control group to no action or to the traditional action.

Thus, medical experiments can only be carried out in a situation of uncertainty. Unfortunately, some potential investigators are so convinced as to the benefits of a treatment or preventive measure, that they are unwilling to carry out a controlled experimental test of its effects. Their *feeling* of certainty, even if based on inadequate evidence, makes them reluctant to withhold the treatment from a control group. Similarly, the unreasonable skeptic, convinced of the value of either the traditional treatment or doing nothing, may be unwilling to try new methods on an experimental basis. Both types of "believers" should realize that the failure to carry out a controlled experiment, when it is needed and feasible, is also unethical (Hill, 1971).

Sensitivity to the ethical aspects of human experimentation has resulted in the formation of committees in universities and other research institutions to review and approve all proposed studies of human subjects. It is now commonly believed that whenever possible, the potential subject should share in the decision as to whether he or she should participate in the study. This decision should be made with adequate understanding of the potential risks and benefits involved. Accordingly, informed consent is generally required from experimental subjects or from appropriate relatives or guardians.

How Experiments Are Carried Out

Experimental epidemiology is concerned primarily with testing the efficacy of measures to *prevent* disease. The preventive measure to be tested is applied to a group of persons. The incidence of the disease or disease-related outcome, such as disability, is measured in this experimental, or treated, group.

In order for the experiment to be informative, it must be controlled; that is, the outcome must be compared to some standard to determine whether any benefit has resulted. The standard may be the outcome in another similar group who do not receive the preventive measure. This control group may, instead, receive either no preventive measure or whatever is currently being applied.

Experiments may involve comparisons among several groups. For example, different amounts or dosages of the treatment may be tested. Or, there may be two or more aspects or elements in a preventive program. In this case, each experimental group may receive a different element or combination of elements. Experiments may even be designed in a more complex fashion so that each group receives a variety of treatments in sequence, possibly including periods of time with no treatment (Smart, 1970).

Randomized Control Groups The traditional and most accepted means of defining the treated and control groups is to identify one large group of all study subjects and then divide them randomly into two or more groups. If only chance determines who gets into one group or another, then the usual tests of statistical significance can be applied, to see whether chance could have produced the observed outcome. Random assignment to groups should be done *after* the subjects are shown to be qualified and willing to participate. This will minimize subsequent losses from one or more groups.

If it is crucial that the treated and control groups be equivalent with regard to certain characteristics that might affect the outcome, the entire study population can be divided, or stratified, into subgroups and each subgroup can then be randomly divided into treated and control subjects. For example, stratification into age subgroups can be accomplished to assure that the treated and control groups have similar age distributions.

If after randomization has taken place, the experimenter would like to be sure that some nonstratified crucial characteristic is similar in the treated and control groups, he should examine the distribution of this characteristic in the two groups. If crucial characteristics differ appreciably, then the experimenter had bad luck in the randomization process. Randomization may have to be repeated, or if not possible, the results of the experiment will have to be analyzed in a way that takes into account the differences in these important characteristics. Appropriate analytic methods are discussed in Chap. 11.

Nonrandom Control Groups Randomized control groups are not always available for epidemiologic experiments. The reason may be economic. Funds may not be adequate for careful follow-up of both a treated and control group of adequate size. Or, the extra assurance that can be provided by this more ideal method may be judged to be not worth the cost involved. Also, there may not be enough subjects available for the two groups.

Even if there are enough subjects and enough money, randomization into subgroups may be impossible or may fail in actual practice. Randomization is impossible if the preventive measure can be applied only to the entire population, as when something is added to the water supply of a total community. Or, learning of the preventive measure through conversations with members of the treated group or through publicity campaigns, the control group may adopt the preventive measure to almost the same extent as does the treated group.

If randomized control groups are not used, alternative standards of comparison are available. A comparison group may be selected from persons known to be similar to the experimental group with respect to several pertinent characteristics such as age, sex, occupation, and social class. Or, if the preventive program is applied to an entire community, a similar untreated community may be used as a control.

Another approach is to have the experimental group serve as its own control. That is, a before-after comparison is made, in which there is a baseline period of observation on the experimental group before any preventive program is applied. The disease experience during this period can be compared with what happens after the program is put into effect.

Even when a separate comparison group is used, a baseline observation period is helpful. If systematic differences between the groups are noted during the baseline period, these can be taken into account in comparing the groups after the preventive measure is applied.

Possible biases or underlying group differences should always be searched for when nonrandom control groups are used. Having a group serve as its own control seems especially attractive, since this appears to eliminate virtually all group differences. However, the control and experimental observations are made during different time periods. Thus, there is the real danger that with the passage of time, other things have happened to the study group leading to the appearance of benefit from the preventive measure when none exists, or conversely, masking true benefits. Rapid changes in diagnostic and treatment methods or even in ways of life are the order of the day; these may result in real or apparent changes in disease incidence that have nothing to do with preventive methods being tested.

Subject Cooperation   Many preventive measures require the cooperation or active participation of the study subjects. Experimental evaluations of these measures must take into account the failure of many subjects to cooperate. Even after initially agreeing to participate, persons drop out of the study for a variety of reasons. Also, in the treated group there will be those who take none or only part of the treatment. Similarly, in the control group there may be some who openly or surreptitiously obtain the treatment on their own.

Study of outcomes should not be limited to the cooperators in each group since they represent a self-selected subgroup, often characterized by higher educational level, higher socioeconomic status, more concern about health and better health habits. Furthermore, if the preventive measure is eventually adopted, it will be applied in the "real world," which also has its full share of noncooperators.

Thus, the most important comparison to be made is of the *entire* study group versus the *entire* control group. This will provide the best estimate of the overall benefit to be obtained from the preventive measure if it is put into practice.

Blind Experiments If possible, experimental subjects should be kept unaware of whether they are treated or control subjects. Then, their own prejudices or enthusiasms will not result in behavior that promotes or inhibits the recognition of disease outcomes. Often, however, the nature of the treatment makes it impossible to keep the subjects "blind" to their assignment to treated or control groups.

More important is that the *assessment* of outcome be blind. Whenever possible, the physicians or others who determine whether the disease outcome has occurred should be unaware of whether the individual is a treated or control subject. The use of objective tests and criteria for diagnosis will help prevent any bias in favor of the treated or control group.

Even when experiments are designed to be blind, the subjects or their evaluators often become aware of their status. If drugs are involved in the treatment, characteristic side effects may reveal their identity. Also, unbeknown to the investigator, medical personnel involved in the care of the subjects may have access to the code or other information which identifies treated and control groups.

Thus, blind experiments are often desired but less often achieved. As for any type of study, careful evaluation of methods and results for possible bias is necessary.

The term "double-blind" is frequently encountered. Some authors use it to refer to experiments where both the assignment to treatment or control group and the assessment of results are blind. Others use it to refer to experiments in which neither the patient nor the physician knows whether the patient is in the experimental or control group.

Sample Size Considerations and Sequential Analysis Statistical methods are available for determining in *advance* how large the treatment and control groups must be, to obtain answers of the desired precision (Ipsen and Feigl, 1970). In general, the more subjects, the greater assurance that the results of the experiment are accurate and not subject to chance variation.

The desirability of having large numbers of subjects is counterbalanced by practical considerations of cost and difficulty. Ethics also enter into decisions about sample size. The more subjects included, the more who will have received the inferior treatment, if either the experimental or control regimen proves to be better.

Sometimes subjects are brought into an experiment over a relatively long period of time rather than all at once. The results for the subjects who started early may be available before the experiment is completed as planned. It is tempting to peek at early results for a few subjects and end the experiment if a difference between experimental and control groups is apparent. Unfortunately, these preliminary findings will not have the accuracy that was originally planned and agreed upon for the experiment. Stopping the experiment at this point may seem economically or ethically justified, but unless the differences noted are striking and compelling, the investigators may later regret reaching a conclusion on the basis of incomplete data. On the other hand, treatment-control differences may be much greater than originally expected, and therefore accurately demonstrable on a small number of subjects. The investigators would certainly not wish to continue the experiment, if they could be sure that this were the case.

Sequential analysis is a relatively new statistical method which allows an experiment to be ended as soon as an answer of the desired precision is obtained. The result of the comparison of each pair of subjects, one treated and one control, is looked at as soon as it becomes available and is added to all previous results. A criterion for deciding in favor of either the experimental or control treatment is specified in advance with the desired degree of accuracy. The comparison of a relatively small number of pairs may show sufficient differences to permit the decision to be reached. If not, the results for each additional pair are added as soon as they become available until the decision criterion is met, or until it becomes apparent that there is no appreciable difference. As soon as any conclusion is reached, the experiment is stopped. The use of sequential analysis in medical experiments is described further by Armitage (1960) and Smart (1970).

Example 1. Controlled Field Trials of Poliomyelitis Vaccine

The first poliomyelitis vaccine that was widely used in the United States was the injectable vaccine containing inactivated virus, developed by Dr. Jonas Salk. By 1953, evidence had accumulated that this vaccine could be safely administered to man and that it stimulated the production of antibody that protected against the three known types of poliomyelitis virus. What was needed next was an experimental trial of the vaccine to demonstrate whether it was safe and effective when put into general use.

A large-scale cooperative field trial was undertaken in 1954, coordinated by the Poliomyelitis Vaccine Evaluation Center at the University of Michigan (Francis et al., 1955). Through the cooperation of state and local health authorities, over 200 areas participated. These were selected partly because they had experienced higher than average poliomyelitis incidence rates in previous years.

The initial plan was to inoculate school children in the second grade and observe the first- and third-graders as a control group. Although this would not permit a blind assessment of outcome, many states had agreed to participate on this basis, and this procedure was carried out in 127 counties or towns in 33 states (called "observed areas"). Eleven states were willing to cooperate in a blind experiment with a randomized control group. In the 84 counties and towns in this latter group (called "placebo areas"), participating children in the first through third grades would all receive a series of three injections, but half would receive the vaccine and half would receive an inactive *placebo*, or *dummy*.

All children in the first through third grades of the participating schools were first identified by means of a "registration form" on which was also recorded birth date, sex, race, and previous history of poliomyelitis or disability. Each child was to give a "participation request" form to his parents. This form described the observed or placebo study and provided space for the parent to sign a request that his child participate in the study. A vaccination record form was used to record all inoculations given to each participant.

Unique identification of each child on all the forms, plus cross-checking and editing of the information was carried out to ensure a high degree of accuracy. In this study there were 200,745 vaccinated and 201,229 receiving placebo among the 1,829,916 first- to third-grade children in the placebo areas, and 221,998 vaccinated second-graders and 725,173 first- and third-grade controls among the 1,080,680 first- to third-graders in the observed areas.

The vaccination phase took place between April 26, 1954 and June 15, 1954. Participating children in each classroom received vaccine or placebo from numbered vials in such a way that all three injections would be of the same material. In the placebo areas, there were vaccinated and placebo children in virtually every class. The vial code numbers could be interpreted as representing vaccine or placebo only at the Evaluation Center. Pre- and post-inoculation blood specimens were obtained from a sample of children to assess antibody response.

During follow-up, through the rest of the year, uniform procedures were instituted to detect and investigate all suspected cases of poliomyelitis among first- through third-grade children, regardless of their participation or vaccination status. The Evaluation Center was notified of all suspected cases plus all deaths from any cause. Each local health department arranged for the complete investigation of each case. The data collected included (1) a complete clinical report including history, physical examination, and spinal fluid findings; (2) laboratory specimens, including stool and blood samples for viral and antibody studies; (3) examinations by a physical therapist to classify the patient according to physical disability; and (4) autopsies, when obtainable for fatal cases.

Checking systems plus a good deal of correspondence with physicians and other persons involved were required to make certain that the data collected were complete. By December 31, 1954 290 case records of the total of 1,103 reported were still incomplete. A campaign of telegrams, telephone calls, letters, and field visits reduced the number of incomplete reports to 78 by the end of January, but the last delinquent report was not received until March 9, 1955.

Criteria were drawn up for interpreting the laboratory and clinical findings, and on the basis of these, the investigated cases were classified as either "not polio," "doubtful polio," "nonparalytic polio," or "paralytic polio." Paralytic cases were further divided into spinal, bulbar, bulbospinal, and fatal. These decisions were all made without knowledge of the vaccination status of the children.

The experiment clearly established the benefits of the vaccines. In the placebo areas the incidence of poliomyelitis was less than half as great in those who were vaccinated (28 per 100,000) as in those who were given placebo (71 per 100,000). Similarly, in the observed areas the incidence was 25 per 100,000 in the vaccinated second-graders and 54 per 100,000 in the first- and third-grade controls. These differences were highly significant statistically. The protection appeared to be only against paralytic poliomyelitis, since there were no appreciable differences between vaccinated and controls in the incidence of nonparalytic disease.

Supporting evidence for the vaccine's effectiveness was obtained from the antibody studies. Furthermore, cases occurring among the vaccinated tended to occur in children who received vaccine which was independently judged less effective, on the basis of antigenic response. Other detailed analyses revealed that the vaccine conferred greater protection against more severe forms of paralysis and that older children appeared to benefit more than younger ones.

No ill effects of the vaccine could be demonstrated. School absenteeism for 6 weeks after the inoculations did not differ significantly among the vaccinated, placebo, and noninoculated populations. Nor was there any difference in the occurrence of rashes or other allergic manifestations, which were very rare despite the presence of small amounts of penicillin in the vaccine and placebo. Other symptoms and illnesses at the time of the injection series were quite unusual and occurred no more often in the vaccinated than in the placebo group. The minute quantities of kidney protein in the vaccine caused some concern about possible side effects on the kidney, but none could be demonstrated in the study, nor could any deaths be reasonably attributed to the vaccine.

This study represents a major achievement in experimental epidemiology. The low incidence of poliomyelitis required that a very large population be studied to provide adequate cases to reliably demonstrate the vaccine's effectiveness. Coordinating a large-scale field trial of this nature is a difficult undertaking. This summary has emphasized study design and data collection efforts, but major problems of a logistical nature should not be forgotten. For example, hundreds of thousands of children all over the country had to be supplied with the right vaccines at the right times, and thousands of blood specimens had to be drawn and transported to 28 different laboratories.

Example 2. Fluoride and Tooth Decay

Experimental studies to test the effects of adding fluorides to community water supplies were begun around 1945. The expectation that raising the fluoride concentration of drinking water to one part per million would safely lower the incidence of tooth decay was based on a number of previous observational studies. These studies had demonstrated that ingestion of water containing large amounts of fluorides during the years of tooth enamel calcification resulted in discoloration and even pitting of the teeth. However, these "mottled" teeth appeared to be quite resistant to decay. Comparisons of dental status in communities with differing fluoride concentrations in their drinking water showed that where the level was about one part per million, the decay rates were relatively low and no disfiguring mottling of the enamel was apparent.

On the basis of these findings the water supply of certain low-fluoride communities was treated on an experimental basis to bring the fluoride concentration up to the desired one-part-per-million concentration. Since randomized control groups could not be obtained for these studies, the experiment was controlled by concurrently measuring dental health status in similar but untreated low-fluoride communities. Furthermore, the dental health of children in the treated communities was assessed before the addition of fluoride, to provide a before-after comparison. Still another comparison was made of each treated community with Aurora, Illinois, where the naturally occurring fluoride concentration in water was 1.2 parts per million and relatively little tooth decay was observed. One of these investigations, the Newburgh-Kingston Caries-Fluorine Study (Dean, 1956, Hilleboe, 1956, Schlesinger et al., 1956, Ast et al., 1956) will be described here.

The cities studied, Newburgh and Kingston, New York are located on the Hudson River about 35 miles apart. Each had a population of about 30,000. Newburgh agreed to serve as the treated community, and beginning May 2, 1945, sodium fluoride was added to its drinking water to raise the fluoride content from about 0.1 part per million to 1.0–1.2 parts per million. Kingston agreed to serve as the control community, and its water supply with a fluoride concentration of about 0.1 part per million was left unchanged.

During the year prior to adding fluoride, baseline dental examinations were carried out on the public and parochial school children, ages 6–12, in both communities. Baseline pediatric examinations were performed on smaller samples. Kingston and Newburgh children were, at first, similar regarding both general health and the prevalence of tooth decay.

Periodic assessments of both dental and other health measures were made subsequently. Although the caries experience in Kingston children remained relatively stable, a continuing improvement was noted in Newburgh.

A final evaluation was carried out after the experiment had gone on for 10 years. Over 2,000 children, ages 6–16 were given dental examinations in each community. They were selected by taking every second school child who was present on the day of the examination. Although the clinical dental examinations were not conducted in a blind fashion, x-rays were taken and were randomized at the state health department so that the interpreters would not know whether they were reading Kingston or Newburgh films.

The data analysis was carried out for separate age groups. The Newburgh subjects, ages 6–9, had used fluoridated water all their lives. The older age groups had been exposed to fluoridation starting at later periods in their dental development, and thus might be expected to show less benefit.

The efficacy of fluoridated water in preventing dental decay was clearly shown in this experiment. One of the indexes of the prevalence of tooth decay was the number of decayed, missing, or filled (DMF) permanent teeth per 100 erupted permanent teeth. For the 6–9-year-olds, this measure was 23.1 in Kingston and 10.0 in Newburgh, a relative reduction of 57 percent of the Kingston rate. The reduction in Newburgh was present in all age groups but was relatively less in older children. Thus the DMF rates in 16-year-olds were 58.9 in Kingston and 34.8 in Newburgh, a relative reduction of 41 percent of the Kingston rate. The Kingston-Newburgh differences were found in both the clinical and x-ray examinations.

Dental-caries prevalence rates in Newburgh and other communities with experimental water fluoridation programs were reduced to levels very similar to those noted in Aurora, Illinois. Thus, artifically fluoridated water was also shown to have the same benefit as observed for the naturally occurring fluoride.

Adverse effects of fluoridation were also looked for. There were no instances of disfiguring dental fluorosis or mottling. About 18 percent of the Newburgh children were found to have questionable or mild fluorosis when examined by an expert trained in detecting the effects of fluoride. The mild changes noted would have been hardly noticeable to the average dentist. On the other hand, 19 percent of children in Kingston had nonfluoride opacities or circular patches in the enamel which would have been obvious even to the untrained eye. These were found in only 8 percent of Newburgh children.

The medical examinations, x-ray estimates of bone maturation, measures of growth and development, eye and ear tests, blood counts, and quantitative studies of urinary excretion of albumin, red blood cells, and casts, all revealed no significant differences between Kingston and Newburgh children. Vital statistics data showed no consistent differences between the two communities in cancer and cardiovascular-renal death rates or in infant mortality, maternal mortality, or stillbirth rates.

These community studies present rather convincing evidence of the benefits of water fluoridation. They illustrate how well-designed preventive medical experiments can be carried out even when randomized control groups are not available.

Example 3: Evaluating the Periodic Multiphasic Health Checkup

An experiment to evaluate the long-term effects of periodic multiphasic health checkups is currently in progress at the Kaiser-Permanente Medical Care Program in northern California. Although the results are only beginning to appear at the time of this writing, this experiment is described to introduce the reader to studies of preventive medical services that go beyond the prevention of single diseases.

It is widely accepted in the United States that annual physical examinations are an important means of maintaining good health. The rationale for annual checkups is that the physician may detect early or asymptomatic disease and initiate treatment before serious consequences develop.

Because of this belief, many persons request and expect annual checkups as part of the medical-care services they receive. Providing checkups to large numbers of patients can consume a substantial proportion of a physician's time—time that might also be used to provide more care of the sick. Because of the growing awareness in this country of the high costs and limitations of physician time and medical care resources, efforts to simplify the checkup are being developed and evaluated. Along these lines, paramedical personnel and automated instruments are being used to assist in examinations in order to save physician time.

Yet the basic question still remains as to just how much overall benefit periodic checkups actually offer. While common sense supports the value of early disease detection and treatment, physicians must also conclude that at least some aspects of checkups (such as listening to the heart and lungs of a young healthy patient every year, year after year) are almost always a waste of time.

The available scientific data on this question are surprisingly limited. A few studies have shown reductions in mortality and in other unfavorable outcomes in groups who received periodic health examinations. However, the comparison groups have not been randomly selected but have been superficially similar populations not receiving examinations. Persons who receive examinations have been shown to be like volunteers and other "cooperators" in that they tend to be more educated, more health-conscious, less prone to smoke cigarettes, and so on. Thus, serious questions can be raised about the comparability of the examined and nonexamined populations in these earlier studies.

In the Kaiser-Permanente experiment, the control group is quite comparable to the examined, or "study," group. Both groups of over 5,000 subjects were selected on the basis of having certain digits in their medical record numbers, a systematic sampling method that is equivalent to random sampling, since these numbers are assigned in sequence with no relationship to any personal characteristics. These two samples were drawn from a large pool of Kaiser Foundation Health Plan members living in Oakland, Berkeley, and San Francisco, California and aged 35–54 when the study started in 1964. To minimize losses to follow-up, another selection criterion for potential study subjects was that they must have been Health Plan members for at least 2 years, since persons quitting the Plan tend to do so soon after joining.

Each study-group subject has been telephoned and urged to have a multiphasic health checkup every year. Control-group subjects have not been urged or reminded to have these checkups, but, of course, they are entitled to receive this service if they so choose. On the average, 20 to 24 percent of the control group have sought this service each year, and during the first 7 years of the study, the average number of examinations received per subject was 1.34, with 47 percent of control members having received none. In contrast, 60 to 70 percent of the urged study group have been examined annually, and the average number of examinations per subject in 7 years was 3.54, with only 17 percent of study group having had no examinations. Thus the urging has resulted in a considerably larger "dosage" of multiphasic checkups for the study group.

Follow-up of the two groups has consisted of a number of components to measure the development of morbidity, mortality, and disability and to assess the utilization and costs of all medical-care services. Hospitalizations and outpatient visits are tabulated, and the names of all persons lost to follow-up are sent to the state health department for a check against death certificate lists to see if they have died. A questionnaire survey is sent to both groups at approximately 2-year intervals to learn of the development of disability and other pertinent problems.

Whenever possible, assessment of various outcomes is made in such a way as to avoid bias in favor of study or control group. For example, even though submitting subjects' recent addresses would help the state health department search for deaths, this is not done, since the annual telephone contact with the study group leads to more accurate and up-to-date information about addresses than is available for the control group.

As mentioned, this study is still in progress. Results in the first 7 years show that the checkup program has had an impact on the discovery and diagnosis of a variety of conditions. The older men in the study group, those aged 45–54 when the experiment started, showed some benefit from these examinations in the form of less disability and time lost from work than was experienced by the older control group men. There also appeared to be some reduction in the study group of mortality from conditions that would be expected to be influenced by early detection and therapy, such as hypertension and its complications. Economically, the added costs of the examinations were more than made up for by the greater earning power of the examined group due to their diminished disability and mortality (Cutler et al., 1973, Ramcharan et al., 1973, Dales et al., 1973, Collen et al., 1973).

REFERENCES

Armitage, P., *Sequential Medical Trials.* (Springfield, Ill.: Charles C Thomas, 1960).

Ast, D. B., D. J. Smith, B. Wachs, and K. T. Cantwell. 1956. Newburg-Kingston caries-fluorine study XIV. Combined clinical and roentgenographic dental findings after 10 years of fluoride experience. *J. Am. Dent. Assoc.*, **52**:314–325.

Collen, M. F., L. G. Dales, G. D. Friedman, C. D. Flagle, R. Feldman, and A. B. Siegelaub. 1973. Multiphasic Checkup Evaluation Study: 4. Preliminary cost benefit analysis for middle aged men. *Preventive Medicine*, **2**:236–246.

Cutler, J. L., S. Ramcharan, R. Feldman, A. B. Siegelaub, B. Campbell, G. D. Friedman, L. G. Dales, and M. F. Collen. 1973. Multiphasic Checkup Evaluation Study: 1. Methods and population. *Preventive Medicine*, **2**:197–206.

Dales, L. G., G. D. Friedman, S. Ramcharan, A. B. Siegelaub, B. A. Campbell, R. Feldman, and M. F. Collen. 1973. Multiphasic

Checkup Evaluation Study: 3. Outpatient clinic utilization, hospitalization and mortality experience after seven years. *Preventive Medicine*, **2**:221–235.

Dean, H. T. 1956. Fluorine in the control of dental caries. *J. Am. Dent. Assoc.*, **52**:1–8.

Francis, T., Jr., R. F. Korns, R. B. Voight, M. Boisen, F. M. Hemphill, J. A. Napier, and E. Tolchinsky. May 1955. An evaluation of the 1954 poliomyelitis vaccine trials: Summary report. *Am. J. Public Health*, **45**:(No. 5, Part 2)1–63.

Hill, A. B., *Principles of Medical Statistics*, 9th ed. (London: Oxford University Press, 1971), Chap. 20.

Hilleboe, H. E. 1956. History of the Newburgh-Kingston caries-fluorine study. *J. Am. Dent. Assoc.*, **52**:291–295.

Hutchison, G. B., Evaluation of preventive measures, in *Preventive Medicine*, edited by D. W. Clark and B. MacMahon (Boston: Little, Brown, 1967), pp. 39–54.

Ipsen, J., and P. Feigl, *Bancroft's Introduction to Biostatistics*, 2d ed., (New York: Harper and Row, 1970), pp. 180–184.

Ramcharan, S., J. L. Cutler, R. Feldman, A. B. Siegelaub, B. Campbell, G. D. Friedman, L. G. Dales, and M. F. Collen. 1973. Multiphasic Checkup Evaluation Study: 2. Disability and chronic disease after seven years of multiphasic health checkups. *Preventive Medicine*, **2**:207–220.

Schlesinger, E. R., D. E. Overton, H. C. Chase, and K. T. Cantwell. 1956. Newburgh-Kingston caries-fluorine study XIII. Pediatric findings after ten years. *J. Am. Dent. Assoc.*, **52**:296–306.

Smart, J. V., *Elements of Medical Statistics*, 2d ed. (London: Staples Press, 1970) Chaps. 5, 8, 10–12.

Chapter 10

Clinical Studies of Disease Outcome

Just as some questions relating to disease occurrence and disease etiology are best answered by studying population groups, clinical problems often require the study of *groups* of patients. Many methods for studying patient groups are similar to the epidemiologic methods for studying populations, discussed in previous chapters.

The process by which healthy people become sick and the factors that determine who will become sick and who will stay healthy are the primary concern of epidemiology. Many clinical studies, on the other hand, aim at sick people and try to identify the factors that determine what the outcome of illness will be. This difference in focus between the two types of studies is illustrated in Fig. 10-1. Note that illness or disease can have several outcomes, including recovery, improvement, no change, worsening, complications, disability, and death.

The ultimate goal of epidemiology is to learn how to prevent

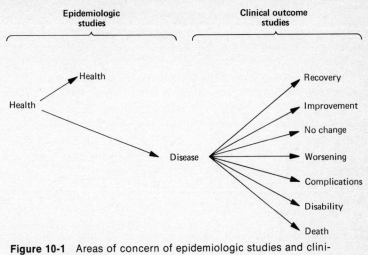

Figure 10-1 Areas of concern of epidemiologic studies and clinical outcome studies.

disease. The ultimate goal of clinical studies is to learn how to cure or successfully treat disease.

The purpose of this chapter is to demonstrate some of the parallels between clinical studies of disease outcome and epidemiologic studies and to describe the analytic methods commonly used to measure disease outcome.

Natural History of Disease

Studies of the *natural history of disease* are analogous to descriptive studies in epidemiology. The outcomes of a particular disease are observed and the proportions of the affected patients developing each outcome are measured. This information is the basis of *prognosis*, that is, predicting a patient's future. As in descriptive epidemiologic studies, disease outcomes are generally determined for major subgroups of patients such as males versus females, various age groups, and so on.

A good example of a study of the natural history of disease is Bland and Jones' (1951) 20-year study of 1,000 children and adolescents with rheumatic fever or chorea. These patients, initially hospitalized at the House of the Good Samaritan in Boston, were carefully followed up into adulthood. Among the findings were that 65 percent of the children had signs of rheumatic heart disease when they recovered from their acute illness, but 16 percent of those with such signs had no evidence of heart disease 20 years later. On the other hand, 44 percent of those without apparent heart disease initially had valvular disease when they were examined as adults. Also described were the recurrence rates of acute rheumatic fever, the evolution of murmurs, and the frequency of deaths and other sequelae of the disease.

Analytic Studies

The clinical investigator usually wishes to go beyond general descriptions of prognosis and to determine what factors lead to improvement, worsening, death, and other outcomes. Such factors include patient characteristics and environmental influences. One of the main environmental factors that is investigated is, of course, therapy.

Analytic clinical investigations of prognostic factors may be carried out in a fashion quite analogous to prevalence, case-control, and incidence studies in epidemiology. A physician is conducting what amounts to an informal prevalence study when he makes rounds on two wards caring for paralyzed stroke patients and notices that in one ward, several patients have decubitus ulcers (bedsores) and on the other, the patients are ulcer-free. He will probably conclude that being on the first ward is conducive to the development of this complication of paralytic stroke and will make some appropriate comments to the nursing staff.

Analytic studies of factors affecting prognosis are usually similar to incidence studies. That is, attributes of the group of patients are assessed early in the course of the illness. Then, the patients are followed up to determine outcome.

The clinical investigator can adopt this prospective follow-up approach much more readily than can the epidemiologist. The rates of development of many disease outcomes are relatively high, compared to the incidence of most diseases in a population. Thus, a relatively small patient group can be observed in one clinic or hospital until the various outcomes are noted.

Consider, for example, the follow-up study by Stahlman et al. (1967) to determine characteristics predicting the outcome of hyaline membrane disease in the newborn. Of 115 affected newborns studied, 33, or 29 percent, died in the neonatal period. A number of measurements taken within 12 hours of birth, such as arterial-blood oxygen tension, birth weight, and respiratory rate, all proved to be related to mortality, and statistical-significance tests showed that these relationships could not reasonably be attributed to chance. Thus, the predictive value of these measurements was demonstrable in this study of only several dozen patients.

Some analytic follow-up studies of prognosis deal with events that develop relatively slowly and infrequently, so that large numbers of patients must be followed for years. This is particularly true of chronic diseases. The Health Insurance Plan of Greater New York (HIP) has been investigating the prognosis of patients with angina pectoris and myocardial infarction. One such study demonstrated a relationship of blood pressure in these patients to the probability of subsequent myocardial infarction and cardiac death—the higher the blood pressure, the worse the prognosis. This study was based on 275 cases of angina pectoris and 881 cases of a first myocardial infarction found among 55,000 men during a 4-year case-finding period. The cases were followed up for 4.5 years (Frank et al., 1972).

When an analytic follow-up study cannot be carried out, it may be practical to use an approach analogous to the case-control method in epidemiology. That is, a group of patients with one particular outcome may be compared with a group showing another outcome, to see whether the two groups differ in any characteristic that might have affected or predicted the outcome. An example is Ellenberg's (1971) study of sexual impotence complicating diabetes mellitus. Forty-five impotent diabetic men ("cases") were compared with thirty male diabetics who were not impotent ("controls"). The potent diabetics were selected to match the impotent group with respect to age distribution and duration of diabetes. The striking difference between the two groups was in the percentage showing evidence of neuropathy affecting the autonomic system—82 percent of the impotent versus 10 percent of the potent. Thus it could be concluded that most cases of impotence in diabetics were due to diabetic neuropathy rather than endocrine or other abnormalities.

Therapeutic Trials

The therapeutic trial is an experiment as applied to clinical medicine. In it, a drug, a surgical operation, or other therapy is applied to patients and the outcome is compared with that observed in a suitable control group.

It is essential that alternative therapies be evaluated in a well-controlled fashion using, whenever possible, the techniques of random allocation and blind assignment and assessment described in Chap. 9. The influence of the therapist's personality and the placebo effect (or tendency of patients to respond favorably even when a drug has no active ingredients) are potent determinants of outcome and should not be allowed to bias the experiment. Furthermore, because of wide variations in the way individual patients respond to treatment, large groups of patients are often required. Large groups will help ensure that an observed relationship between a treatment and an outcome is not due to chance and that the relationship has some general applicability.

The value of large patient series is apt to be forgotten by clinicians working with patients on an individual basis. A physician's use or avoidance of a particular therapy is often guided by his experience with a few patients. His view of the values or dangers of a particular treatment may be exaggerated just because, as luck would have it, the first two or three patients treated happened to respond unusually well or unusually poorly.

There is a widespread belief that the individual physician is the best judge of the value of a drug or other treatment. Through his knowledge of the patient, he may well be the best judge of what is most appropriate for that patient's particular problems. However, the average physician's limited experience with a few patients does not usually provide enough information to state a general principle or conclusion that one therapy is better than another. He may be able to detect dramatic effects such as the value of penicillin versus no antibiotic in treating lobar pneumococcal pneumonia. But conclusions as to less-striking differences between therapies should be based on good-sized and representative series of patients with observations controlled as well as possible.

Medical history is full of examples of therapies which become accepted or popular in an epidemic of enthusiasm based on uncontrolled observations. Feeding this epidemic is the preference of authors and journals for reporting positive findings over negative findings. If the treatment is either not helpful or actually harmful, its use may eventually diminish or end, as its deficiencies become recognized. Unfortunately, during the period of general acceptance, withholding the treatment from some individuals, as is required in a well-controlled experiment, may be considered unethical. Thus it is important to perform a good therapeutic trial as early as possible after the therapy is developed.

Nevertheless, controlled trials are better carried out late than never. For example, the Boston Inter-Hospital Liver Group (BILG) recently completed a well-controlled therapeutic trial which failed to confirm the long-term value of a widely accepted surgical treatment (Resnick et al., 1969). Portacaval-shunt operations had been carried out as an elective prophylactic measure on patients with cirrhosis of the liver to relieve the excess pressure in esophageal varices and prevent serious bleeding episodes. Acceptance of the procedure by the medical profession was based on uncontrolled observations that cirrhotic patients who received this operation did better and lived longer than those who did not. What is often forgotten is that surgeons naturally prefer to operate on the relatively healthy or good-risk patients and reject the poor-risk patients as operative candidates.

In the BILG study, 93 cirrhotic patients with esophageal varices and no prior major bleeding episodes were randomly divided into a surgical and medical group. To avoid selection of the better-risk candidates for shunt surgery in this experiment, each patient was randomly assigned *after* the physicians and surgeons agreed that he or she was a candidate and *after* the patient had consented to have surgery. Both groups were followed up for several years.

The operation apparently did prevent bleeding episodes, as there were significantly more patients with subsequent hemorrhages in the medical group (12/45) than in the surgical group (1/48). However, the mortality of the surgical and medical patients was quite similar. Although the surgical patients were less apt to die of bleeding, they were more apt to die of the hepatorenal syndrome. They were also more prone to develop hepatic encephalopathy.

Another recent controlled therapeutic trial did confirm the value of a much-used but still-debated treatment. For many years, even the individual practitioner could reliably observe that antihypertensive drug therapy brought about a dramatic improvement in the prognosis of severe and malignant hypertension. However the value of drugs for mild to moderate hypertension was less easy to recognize and, until quite recently, was subject to considerable debate. As a result, the Veterans Administration (1967, 1970) carried out a co-operative study in which 523 men with diastolic blood pressures of 90 to 129 mm Hg were assigned randomly to active drug therapy or placebo. Before random assignment there was a trial period during which the potentially uncooperative subjects—those who did not attend clinic regularly or take at least 90 percent of a marked placebo—could be eliminated. (Because most hypertensives feel well, there is little immediate gratification for them in following a regular therapeutic program.)

Therapeutic benefit to the drug-treated group was apparent after only 20 months of follow-up of those starting with diastolic levels of 115 to 129 mm Hg. Only 1 of 73 treated patients developed a major cardiovascular-renal complication, as compared to 27 of 70 control subjects, of whom 4 died. One other treated patient exhibited drug toxicity and had to be removed from the study therapy.

Longer follow-up of more subjects was required to demonstrate benefits of treating milder hypertension—90 to 114 mm Hg diastolic pressure. A total of 380 patients were followed up for an average of 3.3 years. Major complications were observed in 56 of 194 controls, as compared to only 22 of 186 treated subjects. Some complications, such as stroke, showed a markedly lower incidence among the treated group.

Concomitant with the reporting of controlled observations such as these has been a growing awareness that hypertension is serious, and that large numbers of persons in this country are hypertensive and not aware of it. Moreover, many persons who are aware of hypertension are not being treated adequately or consistently. Thus the detection and sustained treatment of hypertension may become a major public health effort in the near future.

Commonly Used Measures of Disease Outcome

Rates   Just as incidence rates are used in epidemiology to measure the development of disease in healthy persons, the outcomes of illness can be measured similarly in groups of sick persons. Thus one may speak of recovery rates, disability rates, death rates, and so on, referring to the proportion of the ill that recover, become disabled, or die per unit of time. Again, the proportion of the sick who manifest a particular outcome at one point in time is analogous to a point prevalence rate of disease in a general population.

Survival   Measures of mortality outcome are often expressed in terms of *survival* rather than death. For comparative purposes, it is not particularly important whether one focuses on successes or failures. However, the data from clinical studies are so often analyzed and presented in terms of survival that it is desirable to be familiar with the approaches used. It should be remembered, also, that these measures need not be restricted to life and death. They can be applied to any mutually exclusive alternatives. Thus, in a study of the development of congestive heart failure in cardiac patients, remaining free of failure can be considered analogous to survival.

One of the most common measures of outcome is the proportion surviving for a particular duration. Any duration may be chosen—5 years is frequently used in studies of the surgical treatment of cancer, because for many types of cancer, if a patient survives for 5 years it is likely that he has been cured. Thus the "5-year survival rate" or "5-year cure rate" merely refers to that proportion of the original patient group still alive after 5 years of follow-up.

Another measure of survival that has been used is the "mean duration of survival." As mentioned in Chap. 2, page 19, the mean duration should be used for comparative purposes only when all patients have died. When some are still living, it is preferable to compare *median duration of survival* or some other *quantile* of *survival durations* because once the stated percentage have died, their survival cannot change. For example, after 75 out of 100 patients have died, the survival duration of the seventy-fifth person becomes the 75th percentile of survival durations for the entire group. This cannot change no matter how much longer the other 25 live. The mean, on the other hand, is not finally determined until all 100 have died.

One of the most common and probably the most informative measures of survival is the survival curve. Starting initially at 100 percent, it shows the proportion still surviving at each subsequent point in time for as long as information is available. Fig. 10-2 shows the curves for the medical and surgical patients in the BILG study of portacaval shunt. The similarity in their survival experience is apparent.

Another graph, Fig. 10-3, shows marked differences in survival for several subgroups of patients with scleroderma, from the study by Medsger et al. (1971). The proportions of scleroderma patients surviving at the end of each year after entry into the study are shown by solid black circles. Those who had no involvement of their lungs,

Figure 10-2 Survival of surgical and medical patients in the Boston Inter-Hospital Liver Group's controlled therapeutic trial of portacaval shunt surgery for esophageal varices. *(Reproduced, by permission, from Resnick et al., 1969.)*

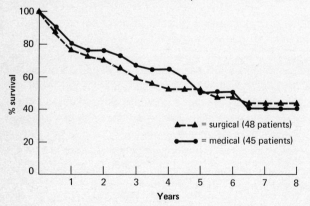

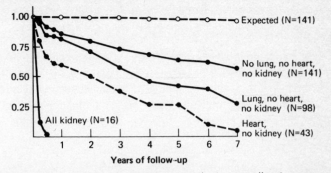

Figure 10-3 Survival of scleroderma patients according to organ involvement. Ordinate shows proportion surviving. *(Reproduced, by permission, from Medsger et al., 1971.)*

heart, or kidneys did the best, with 56 percent still alive after 7 years. Subgroups with poorer survival were next, those with lung involvement; then, those with heart involvement; and finally, those with kidney involvement, all of whom died within the first half year. For comparison, the expected survival curve is shown on top with clear circles. This is the survival that would have been expected for a group of this age, sex, and racial composition if the overall United States mortality rates for the study years had been applicable.

Construction of survival curves for a certain duration following a specific event or time does not require that all patients be observed for that entire duration. Consider an example in which persons are to be followed for 10 years starting at the time their disease was first diagnosed. The experience of a person who moves away and is lost to follow-up after 5 years is still useful in determining survival rates for the first 5 years. Similarly, someone who is diagnosed and enters the study 1 year before the date that follow-up observations are to be completed contributes to those persons observed during the first year after diagnosis.

Thus, all persons who are observed during each unit of time measured from the starting event can contribute their experience to the survival-rate computation for that time unit. The so-called *actuarial* or *life-table* method takes advantage of all these observations by computing survival rates for each time unit and combining these rates together into one composite survival curve. For details as to methods, which are not difficult to carry out, see Berkson and Gage (1950), Cutler and Ederer (1958), or Hill (1971).

Importance of Starting Times When survival curves (or mortality rates) of two groups are to be compared, it is important that both have the same starting point. The starting time may be placed at the onset of symptoms, the first diagnosis, the beginning of therapy, discharge from a hospital, or some other landmark in the course of the disease.

Failure to follow this principle has led to many conflicting claims and erroneous conclusions as to benefits of therapy. For example, two equally good surgical treatments will appear to have different results if survival is measured from the hospital discharge date for one, and from the date of operation for the other. Measuring from date of discharge excludes operative and immediate postoperative mortality.

Although the inclusion or exclusion of operative mortality makes for an obvious error, more subtle and hard-to-recognize biases may result when follow-up of two groups does not begin at strictly comparable times. Consider a study to evaluate the efficacy of a new procedure for the early diagnosis of a disease. Even if detecting the disease early does not prolong life, it might appear to do so if survival is measured from the date of *early* diagnosis instead of from the usual diagnosis date resulting from traditional methods. Procedures for overcoming this bias are discussed by Feinleib and Zelen (1969).

Similarly, treatment measures for rapidly fatal diseases may appear more effective than they really are if they are initiated after a short delay. Part of the apparent improvement in in-hospital mortality from myocardial infarction, experienced by patients in coronary-care units, may be related to the fact that many heart attack victims die shortly after the onset of the attack. As noted by Kodlin, patients in coronary-care units have already survived the short delay between admission to the hospital and admission to the unit.

REFERENCES

Berkson, J., and R. P. Gage. 1950. Calculation of survival rates for cancer. *Proc. Staff Meet. Mayo Clinic*, **25**:270–286.

Bland, E. F., and T. D. Jones. 1951. Rheumatic fever and rheumatic heart disease: A twenty-year report on 1,000 patients followed since childhood. *Circulation*, **4**:836–843.

Cutler, S. J., and F. Ederer. 1958. Maximum utilization of the life table method in analyzing survival. *J. Chron. Dis.* **8**:699–712.

Ellenberg, M. 1971. Impotence in diabetes: The neurologic factor. *Ann. Intern. Med.*, **75**:213–219.

Feinleib, M., and M. Zelen. 1969. Some pitfalls in the evaluation of screening programs. *Arch. Environ. Health*, **19**:412–415.

Frank, C. W., E. Weinblatt, S. Shapiro, and R. Sager. 1972. Prognosis of men with coronary heart disease as related to blood pressure. *Circulation*, **38**:432–438.

Hill, A. B.: *Principles of Medical Statistics*, 9th ed. (London: Oxford University Press, 1971), pp. 228–236.

Kodlin, D. On the status of coronary care unit statistics. To be submitted for publication.

Medsger, T. A., A. T. Masi, G. P. Rodnan, T. G. Benedek, and H. Robinson. 1971. Survival with systemic sclerosis (Scleroderma): A life-table analysis of clinical and demographic factors in 309 patients. *Ann. Intern. Med.*, **75**:369–376.

Resnick, R. H., T. C. Chalmers, A. M. Ishihara, A. J. Garceau, A. D. Callow, E. M. Schimmel, E. T. O'Hara, and the Boston Inter-Hospital Liver Group. 1969. A controlled study of the prophylactic portacaval shunt: A final report. *Ann. Intern. Med.*, **70**:657–688.

Stahlman, M. T., E. J. Battersby, F. M. Shepard, and W. J. Blankenship: 1967. Prognosis in hyaline-membrane disease: use of a linear-discriminant. *New Engl. J. Med.*, **276**:303–309.

Veterans Administration Cooperative Study Group on Antihypertensive Agents. 1967. Effects of treatment on morbidity and mortality: results in patients with diastolic blood pressures averaging 115 through 129 mm. Hg. *J. Am. Med. Assoc.*, **202**:1028–1034.

Veterans Administration Cooperative Study Group on Antihypertensive Agents. 1970. II. Results in patients with diastolic blood pressure averaging 90 through 114 mm. Hg. *J. Am. Med. Assoc.*, **213**:1143–1152.

Chapter 11

Making Sense out of Statistical Associations

Positive findings of epidemiologic or clinical outcome studies are usually referred to as statistical associations. It is essential to have a proper perspective of the meaning and importance of statistical associations. All too frequently they are under- or overinterpreted. With regard to smoking, for example, those at one extreme discount the strong epidemiologic evidence relating cigarette smoking and lung cancer as being "only statistical." At the other extreme are those who quickly blame a whole host of health problems on cigarettes on the basis of weak epidemiologic evidence, without considering the possible role of other important characteristics of persons who smoke.

Statements and Measures of Statistical Association

In discussing the various types of epidemiologic and related studies in Chaps. 5 through 10, the usual methods of expressing the results of these studies have been mentioned several times. Typically, the findings would be that persons having one characteristic or environmental exposure have a higher or lower incidence or prevalence of a disease than persons with a different characteristic or exposure. Or, the association may be expressed in terms of a greater or lesser proportion of the characteristic in the diseased as compared to the nondiseased. Similar statements may express the fact that there is an association between one characteristic and another, or between one disease and another.

In addition to these easily understood statements of association in terms of differences in rates or proportions, epidemiologists sometimes employ other statistical tools to measure and describe associations. For example, data may suggest that there is a linear relationship between two quantitative variables. In a perfect linear relationship, for every unit of increase in one variable the other increases or decreases proportionally. One useful measure of association, the correlation coefficient, indicates the degree to which a set of observations fits a linear relationship. (For method of computation and more discussion, see Hill, 1971, Chaps. 15 and 16 or Ipsen and Feigl, 1970, Chap. 9.) This coefficient, often represented by the letter r, can vary between $+1$ and -1. If $r = +1$, there is a perfect linear relationship in which one variable varies directly with the other. If $r = 0$, there is no association between the variables. If $r = -1$, there is again a perfect association, but one variable varies inversely with the other.

Plotted on a graph showing the relationship between two variables, data points would follow a slanted straight line if the correlation coefficient is $+1$ or -1. Where there is some, but not complete, correlation, the data points would not fall into line but would appear to cluster about a line. If there is no correlation at all, data points would form a regular or irregular clump with no underlying slanted line apparent. Note that the data points for the states in Fig. 11-1 show some degree of linear relationship between cigarettes sold per capita and coronary-heart-disease death rates. The correlation coefficient is $+0.55$.

Other methods of measuring associations are also used, but as mentioned, differences in rates or proportions are most commonly employed. Regardless of how a statistical association is measured or expressed, the same problems of interpretation apply.

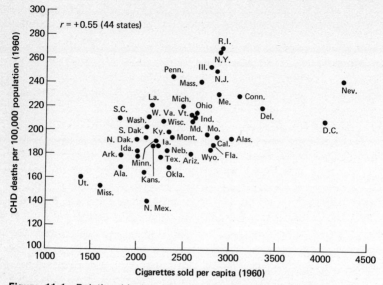

Figure 11-1 Relationship between the age-adjusted total death rate for coronary heart disease and per capita cigarette consumption in 44 states in 1960. *(Reproduced, by permission, from Friedman, 1967.)*

Associations Based on Groups of Groups

It has been emphasized in this book that, in epidemiology, the group is the unit of concern. Groups that provide the most useful and relevant information are *groups of individuals.* Nevertheless, it is also possible to study *groups of groups.* Statistical associations found in groups of groups may be useful, but they may also be quite misleading and not at all applicable to the individuals within the groups.

Consider, for example, the data shown in Fig. 11-1, relating per capita cigarette consumption to coronary-heart-disease mortality rates in 44 states in 1950. The statistical association shown graphically and by the correlation coefficient of +0.55, involves a group of states rather than a group of persons. Although the findings are suggestive of an association between cigarette smoking and coronary-heart-disease mortality in persons, we cannot be sure from these data alone that the persons who smoked in these states truly experienced a higher coronary heart disease mortality rate. (Actually, the association between smoking and coronary heart disease death rates had already been shown in groups of individuals when the study yielding Fig. 11-1 was done. This study's purpose was to cast some light on the striking geographic variation in coronary mortality in the United States.)

The potential for drawing fallacious conclusions about groups of individuals from associations observed in groups of groups was emphasized by Robinson (1950), who termed the latter "ecological correlations." He noted, for example, that among *persons* age 10 and over in the United States there was a moderate *positive* association between being foreign-born and being illiterate. However, looked at on the basis of *geographic regions* (i.e., groups), there was a stronger *negative* correlation. That is, those regions with the lowest percentages of population foreign-born had the highest percentages who were illiterate. Thus a conclusion about the relationship of nativity to literacy based solely on a study of geographic units would have been quite misleading.

Most epidemiologic observations showing that geographic differences in disease rates parallel geographic differences in possible causative factors are associations involving groups of groups. The same may be said of parallel time trends. As such, these correlations in space and time are interesting clues, but their limitations should be recognized. Failure of investigators to respect the possible fallacies involved has contributed to the mistrust of statistics as exemplified by Disraeli's famous reference to "lies, damn lies, and statistics."

Evaluating Statistical Associations Involving Groups of Individuals

Fortunately, the main body of epidemiologic knowledge involves associations found in groups of individuals. When these associations emerge from a study, four basic questions usually require immediate attention:

1 Could the association have been observed just by chance?

2 Could other variables have accounted for the observed relationship?
3 To whom does the association apply?
4 Does the association represent a cause-and-effect relationship?

Evaluating the Possible Role of Chance

Regarding the first question, we have already mentioned in Chap. 3, page 25, that chance plays a role in determining the outcome of a study. The fewer the subjects, the more the observations may be influenced by chance sampling variation. Statistical significance tests are used to determine the probability that the observed association could have occurred by chance alone, if no association really exists. Selecting the appropriate test depends on the nature of the data and the method by which they are analyzed. For example, if the data analysis results in a fourfold table with subjects classified by presence or absence of a trait and of disease as illustrated by Table 3-2, page 39, the chi square test may be most appropriate. Comparing the mean level of a quantitative attribute in a disease group with the mean level in a control group may involve a "t" test of the difference between two means. The reader is referred to medical-statistics texts such as Hill (1971, Chaps, 11–14) or Ipsen and Feigl (1970, Chaps. 6, 8) for further details.

Unfortunately, the word "significant" in "statistically significant" is often misinterpreted as representing the medical or biological significance of an association. A slight difference in the mean hemoglobin concentration between two groups such as 0.1 gm/100 ml may be statistically significant if the two groups are large—that is, it is most unlikely to be due to chance. However this difference may be totally unimportant for health or longevity, or in relation to a disease under investigation. Thus, to say that one group's mean level is significantly lower than that of the other group has connotations that should be avoided by stressing the fact that *statistical* and not *biological* significance is being discussed.

Evaluating the Role of Other Variables

Ruling out chance as a likely explanation is only the first step in making sense out of an association. Equally, if not more, important is to attempt to rule out other variables as possible explanations for the association. To show in a very simple way how a third variable may account for part or all of a statistical association, an imaginary set of data is graphically plotted in Fig. 11-2. The figure shows, let us say, degree of coronary atherosclerosis measured by coronary angiography as related to hand-grip strength. Note that all eight data points form a pattern, showing an association between the two variables. That is, on the average, those with stronger grips tend to have more coronary atherosclerosis.

However, also note that four of the data points are shown by open circles and four by solid black circles. The open circles happen to represent four women and the black circles, four men. Looking at each sex group separately by covering the other four points, it can be seen that there is no relationship between grip strength and amount of atherosclerosis. It is only because the two sexes have been combined in one set of data that the association appears. Thus, sex difference constitutes a third underlying variable that completely explains the apparent association between grip strength and coronary atherosclerosis, which is therefore considered a *spurious* or *secondary* association.

Another set of fictitious data, shown in Table 11-1, again

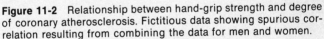

Figure 11-2 Relationship between hand-grip strength and degree of coronary atherosclerosis. Fictitious data showing spurious correlation resulting from combining the data for men and women.

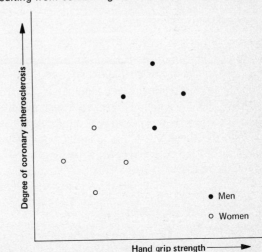

Table 11-1   Relationship between Parental Death and Low-Back Pain History. Fictitious Data Showing Spurious Association Due to Relation of Both Variables to Age.

Age	Total number	History of low-back pain	
		Number	Percent
30–39			
All subjects	200	20	10
Any parent dead	100	10	10
No parent dead	100	10	10
40–49			
All subjects	200	40	20
Any parent dead	140	28	20
No parent dead	60	12	20
50–59			
All subjects	200	60	30
Any parent dead	180	54	30
No parent dead	20	6	30
Total, all ages			
All subjects	600	120	20
Any parent dead	420	92	22
No parent dead	180	28	16

illustrates how an underlying variable, age, can result in an apparent association between two other variables when no real association exists. A total of 600 persons, ages 30–59, were asked whether they have ever been troubled by low-back pain and whether their parents were still living or whether either their mother or father had died.

The top section of the table shows the findings for the 200 subjects in their thirties. Twenty, or 10 percent, reported low-back pain. Also, half had both parents living and half reported at least one parent dead. Of the 100 in either parental-survival group, 10, or 10 percent, reported low-back pain. Thus, in this subgroup, death of a parent was not related to low-back pain.

The next section of the table shows the results for 200 subjects in their forties. At this later age a larger proportion had lost a parent ($^{140}/_{200}$), and a larger proportion reported low-back pain (20 percent), but parental death was again not related to low-back pain. In either parental survival group, 20 percent reported low-back pain.

The results for 200 subjects in their fifties also showed no relationship between the two study variables. The proportion with at least one dead parent was still higher ($^{180}/_{200}$), and the prevalence of a low-back-pain history was higher (30 percent) but again, the 30 percent low-back-pain prevalence held true for subjects both with and without a parent dead.

Now, look at what happens when the data for the three age groups are simply added together, as shown at the bottom of the table. A total of 22 percent of patients with a parent dead report low-back pain, whereas only 16 percent with both parents living have this complaint. The data for all ages combined appear to show that parental loss *is* related to low-back pain, whereas we know that in any age decade this is not the case.

The apparent relationship of low-back pain to parental loss in the total group is attributable to the difference in age distribution between those with and without a dead parent. Stated simply, those with a dead parent contain a higher proportion of older people and, therefore, are more apt to report low-back pain. Actually, 180, or 43 percent, of the 420 subjects with at least one parent dead were in their fifties, whereas only 20, or 11 percent, of the 180 subjects with no parents dead were in their fifties.

Handling Spurious Associations Due to Related Variables

Prevention   Knowledge of previous epidemiologic findings or of the pathophysiology of the disease under investigation will often suggest related variables that may produce a spurious association. A study may be designed and carried out so as to prevent these related variables from producing misleading group differences. For example, cases and controls may be matched for age so that differences in age distribution will not lead to spurious associations such as the one described above.

It may not be possible to "control" all pertinent variables in this manner at the outset. Also, underlying variables may come to light or be thought of later, when the data are being analyzed. Fortunately, it is possible to analyze data in ways that take into account or control extraneous variables.

Specification The simplest method for controlling variables in the data analysis is *specification.* This involves examining the data separately for each subgroup of subjects who fall into one particular category or level of the variable to be controlled. In the above example involving a relationship between hand-grip strength and coronary atherosclerosis, the fact that the correlation is spurious and due to sex differences becomes obvious if we *specify* sex and look at the data separately for men and women. Similarly, if the parental-loss–back-pain association is examined in specific age groups, it is no longer apparent.

Actually, age and sex are so often related to disease occurrence and to other variables that it is customary to examine data in specific age-sex subgroups before combining them into an overall tabulation. This standard approach to data analysis in epidemiology is probably the reason that an epidemiologist has been defined as "a physician broken down by age and sex."

Just as specification can show associations to be spurious, it can also be used to show that suspected underlying variables are not explanations for an association. For example, in a study of smoking and the leukocyte count (Friedman et al., 1973), it was suspected that higher mean leukocyte counts in smokers than in nonsmokers might really be due to chronic bronchitis, which is related both to smoking and to the leukocyte count. The data were analyzed separately for persons with and without evidence of chronic bronchitis. When this was done, large smoker-nonsmoker differences in mean leukocyte count were still present in each subgroup and were, thus, not attributable to chronic bronchitis.

Adjustment Sometimes an investigator would like to compare two or more overall groups, knowing that they differ in a pertinent third variable. It is possible, by means of a procedure known as *adjustment*, to make such comparisons, controlling for differences in an extraneous variable. For example, in evaluating the parental-loss–back-pain association, it is possible through *age-adjustment* to remove the effect of age as a "confounding" variable and compare subjects with and without parental loss to see if either group has a higher prevalence of a low-back-pain history.

Age adjustment by the *direct* method involves choosing a standard population and applying the rates observed for subjects in each specific age category to the corresponding members of the standard population. The choice of a standard population is fairly arbitrary. Often it is the population of a country at a particular time, such as the United States in 1960. Or, frequently, it is the total population involved in the study in question. Or, it may be one particular subgroup of that study population. In our low-back-pain study, for example, one might age-adjust the rates observed in the subgroup with no parental loss, to the subgroup with loss of a parent, or age-adjust the rates of both subgroups to the total study group.

To illustrate how this is accomplished, Table 11-2 shows the direct age adjustment of the rate of low-back pain in the subgroup without parental loss, to the total study population used as a standard. The rate observed in each age category of the subjects with no parental loss is multiplied by the number of subjects in the same age category in the standard population. This yields the number that would be observed in the standard population if the low-back pain rates in the group with no parental loss were applicable to the standard population. The numbers that would be observed in each age group of the standard population are then added together and the total is divided by the total number in the standard population, yielding the age-adjusted rate of 20 percent. In this example, the same age-specific rates of low-back pain were observed in the subjects with parental loss; therefore the age-adjusted rate for this subgroup would also be 20 percent. Thus, using age-adjusted rates, we would correctly conclude that parental loss was not related to low-back pain.

The *indirect* method of age-adjustment is somewhat different from the direct method. Instead of applying the study subgroup's age-specific rates to a standard population, the age-specific rates of the standard population are applied to the corresponding portions

Table 11-2   Example of Direct Age Adjustment: Observed Low-Back Pain Rates Applied to Standard Population Consisting of All Study Subjects

Age	Observed low-back-pain rate	×	Total number in age subgroup of standard population	=	Number that would be observed in standard population
30–39	10%		200		20
40–49	20%		200		40
50–59	30%		200		60
			Total 600		120

$$\text{Age-adjusted rate} = {}^{120}/_{600} = 20\%$$

of the study subgroup. This procedure yields the numbers of cases that would be expected in the study subgroup if the age-specific rates in the standard population had been operative in the study subgroup. The overall expected rate in the study subgroup is then compared to the overall rate in the standard population. Any difference must be attributable to the difference between the age distribution of the subgroup and that of the standard population.

The study subgroup's overall observed rate is then corrected proportionally to make up for this difference in age distribution. For example, if the standard population's overall rate is 80 percent of the expected rate in the study subgroup, then the observed rate in the subgroup is reduced, by multiplying it by 80 percent. After the overall rates in various subgroups have been modified in this manner, they can then be compared fairly with one another. More detailed examples of age adjustment by the direct and indirect methods are given by Hill (1971, Chap. 17).

Indirect adjustment is preferable to direct when there are small numbers in age-specific groups. Rates used in direct adjustment would be based on these small numbers and would thus be subject to substantial sampling variation. With indirect adjustment the rates are more stable since they are based on a large standard population. Note that the expected rate or the expected number of cases, computed by the indirect method, is used in the ratio of observed/expected which constitutes the morbidity (or mortality) ratio described in Chap. 2.

It must be remembered that an age-adjusted rate is an artificial rather than an actual rate. Its value is that it permits one population to be compared with another, with age "controlled." It should not be used if what is wanted is not a comparison, but an accurate description of a population. The age-adjusted rate is a convenient summary of age-specific rates. The age-specific rates themselves are most informative and should be compared whenever possible.

This discussion of adjustment has focused on age adjustment because age is the variable that is most commonly controlled in this manner. However, direct or indirect adjustment may be applied to any variable suspected of playing a role in an association between two study variables.

Other methods More complex statistical procedures are also available for removing the effects of extraneous variables on statistical associations. These procedures involve the more traditional methods such as analysis of covariance, multiple correlation and multiple regression, and discriminant analysis. (The reader with some background in statistics may wish to refer to Morrison, 1967, for further discussion.) Newer methods of multivariate analysis have also been developed for epidemiologic studies of specific diseases.

These techniques are sometimes useful when it is apparent that several factors are not only associated with a disease but also with one another and one wishes to assess the relationship of each factor to the disease, independently of the other factors. An interesting example for the statistically minded reader is the multiple logistic method of Truett et al. (1967), as applied to coronary heart disease.

Although these methods appear to have definite value for certain epidemiologic studies, they all rest on assumptions. These assumptions must be understood by the user because they might or might not apply to the disease and other variables under investigation. Unfortunately, there has been a recent tendency to thoughtlessly throw some data into a computer together with a "canned" multivariate analysis program, expecting that the coefficients and other numbers that come out will somehow reveal a new secret of life. It must be stressed that no method of analysis, no matter how mathematically sophisticated, will substitute for careful evaluation of data based on good scientific judgment and knowledge of the disease process being studied.

General Applicability of an Association

In evaluating observed statistical associations one must always consider to whom they apply. The study in which the association is observed was conducted on a finite group of persons with certain characteristics. Would the association also hold true for other groups? Obviously, the more different groups that show the association, the more certain one can be that it is widely applicable. Where a variety of studies are lacking, it becomes a matter of judgment to determine whether an association observed in one group is applicable to another.

Questions of generality might be raised, for example, regarding the association between serum cholesterol level and coronary heart disease found in the Framingham Study. The study population is virtually all white. Thus it can legitimately be asked whether the same association holds true for blacks and Orientals. Fortunately, other studies provide a positive answer to this question.

More subtle is the fact the Framingham and other similar studies have as subjects volunteers or cooperative people. Does the cholesterol/coronary disease association apply also to uncooperative individuals? While volunteers do differ from others in certain characteristics, it is difficult to imagine that these characteristics would produce this observed relationship. Thus, one might reasonably judge that cholesterol is related to coronary heart disease in the uncooperative as well.

Statistical Associations and Cause-and-Effect Relationships

It is common knowledge that statistical associations do not necessarily imply causation. The "price of tea in China" is a frequently cited example of a variable which can be related statistically to some other variable but has no causal relation to it.

Statistical associations derived from well-controlled experimental studies can usually be interpreted to represent cause-and-effect relationships. Something is done and a result is observed. In epidemiology, however, most studies are observational, and an experiment to establish a cause-and-effect relationship may be difficult or impossible to carry out. Vital decisions affecting public health and preventive medicine must be made on the basis of observational evidence. It is important, therefore, to have some basis for deciding whether or not a statistical association derived from an observational study represents a cause-and-effect relationship.

A number of authors have grappled with this philosophical problem. Certain criteria seem to be universally accepted, while others remain controversial. The reader wishing to explore this question in greater depth should refer to Chap. 2 of MacMahon and Pugh (1970), Chap. 24 of Hill (1971), Yerushalmy (1962), Larsen and Silvette (1968), and Susser (1973).

Strength of the Association In general, the stronger the association the more likely it represents a cause-and-effect relationship. Weak associations often turn out to be spurious and explainable by some known, or as yet unknown, third variable. In order for a strong association to be spurious, the underlying factor that explains it must have an even stronger relation to the disease (Bross, 1966). It is likely, although not certain, that the underlying variable with this even stronger relationship to the disease would be recognizable.

Strength of an association can be measured by the *relative risk*, or the ratio of the disease rate in those with the factor to the rate in those without. The relative risk of lung cancer in cigarette smokers as compared to nonsmokers is on the order of 10:1, whereas the relative risk of coronary heart disease is about 1.5:1. This difference suggests that cigarette smoking is more likely to be a causal factor for lung cancer than for coronary heart disease.

Time Sequence In a causal relationship the characteristic or event associated with the disease must *precede* the disease. This time relationship should be clear in incidence studies. In prevalence and case-control studies it may not always be obvious which came first.

Consistency with Other Knowledge If the association makes sense in terms of known biological mechanisms or other epidemiologic knowledge, it becomes more plausible as a cause-and-effect relationship. Part of the attractiveness of the hypothesis that a high–saturated fat, high-cholesterol diet predisposes to atherosclerosis is the fact that a biologic mechanism can be invoked. Such a diet increases blood lipids which may in turn be deposited in arterial walls. A correlation between the number of telephone poles in a country and its coronary heart disease mortality rate lacks plausibility as a cause-and-effect relationship partly because it is difficult to imagine a biological mechanism whereby telephone poles result in atherosclerosis.

Failure to Find Other Explanations   When a statistical association is observed, the thoughtful investigator will consider possible explanations for the relationship *other* than the observed variable's causing the disease. The data already collected may be used to learn whether these other possible explanations might hold true. Or, additional data may have to be obtained to answer such questions.

Failure to find an alternative to the cause-and-effect hypothesis despite conscientious searching does not prove that there is no alternative. But it does strengthen the evidence for a cause-and-effect relationship.

An interesting example of a search for other explanations comes from a case-control study showing an association between oral contraceptives and thromboembolic disease (Vessey and Doll, 1968). Since it is easy to overlook the diagnosis of deep-vein thrombosis or pulmonary embolism, the investigators considered the possibility that a history of oral-contraceptive use would alert the physician to these conditions, resulting in a spurious association. They reasoned that a spurious association of this type would be strongest among patients with the least evident disease, since this group would contain women whose condition was diagnosed only because they were known to have taken oral contraceptives. Cases were therefore classified by degree of certainty as to the presence of thromboembolism. It was found that the association with oral-contraceptive use was actually less marked among the less certain and milder cases than among the definite and severe cases. Thus, this alternative explanation could reasonably be rejected, lending greater credence to the idea that thromboembolism was actually caused by oral contraceptives.

Other Criteria The criteria listed below have been stressed by some authorities but to this author they seem less valuable as yardsticks for assessing a cause-and-effect relationship per se.

Gradient of Risk It has been stated that if there appears to be a dose-response relationship, this argues for a cause-and-effect relationship. For example, the fact that moderate cigarette smokers have a lung cancer death rate intermediate between nonsmokers and heavy smokers is considered evidence that cigarette smoking causes lung cancer.

This criterion would appear less satisfactory. Threshold phenomena are well known in nature, whereby no effect is seen until a causal stimulus reaches a certain level, above which a response is seen. In this situation a gradient of response might well be absent if two different dosages of the causal factor are well below the threshold level. Conversely, a spurious correlation could easily show a nice gradient. A spurious correlation of cigarette smoking with a disease caused by alcohol consumption might show an apparent dose-response relationship of disease incidence to amount smoked, due to a correlation between amount smoked and amount of alcohol consumed.

Consistency in Several Studies Finding the same association in several different studies provides assurance that the association *exists* and is not an artifact based on the way one particular study was carried out or based on an unusual group of study subjects. In this sense, consistency across studies is reassuring; but it does not argue strongly that an association is one of cause and effect.

Specificity By specificity is meant that the possible causal factor is observed to be associated with one or just a few diseases or effects, rather than a wide variety of diseases. One of the arguments that has been used against cigarette smoking as a cause of lung cancer is that in epidemiologic studies, smoking also appears to be associated with an assortment of seemingly unrelated diseases such as coronary heart disease, peptic ulcer, bladder cancer, and cirrhosis of the liver. It is argued either that smokers differ biologically from nonsmokers in a way that leads health to break down in a variety of ways or that these studies must have been affected by some kind of hidden bias or artifact that falsely incriminates smoking in so many ways.

Although it *is* reassuring when specificity is found, and an apparent lack of specificity *should* lead to some suspicion of an artifact, the importance of a lack of specificity as negative evidence has been overemphasized. This can be readily seen when one considers other recognized disease agents such as the tubercle bacillus and applies the lack of specificity argument to them. How, it might have been asked, can the tubercle bacillus cause an increased rate of lung lesions when it also has been associated with scrofula, meningitis, collapsed vertebrae, peritonitis, bleeding from the kidney, marked wasting, and so on. We now know that the tubercle bacillus can produce a variety of effects, and we have some understanding of the mechanisms by which these occur. Cigarette smoke has a variety of active constituents that get carried throughout the body, so that a lack of specificity is not surprising.

Statistical Associations between Diseases

Epidemiologic and clinical studies may reveal statistical associations between two or more diseases. Two diseases are associated in a population if the incidence or prevalence of one disease is higher when the other is present than when it is absent.

A true association between diseases may occur because one disease predisposes to another (e.g., diabetes mellitus and coronary heart disease) or because both diseases share a common etiologic factor (head injuries and cirrhosis of the liver, both due to alcoholism). Thus, discovery of disease associations may provide valuable information if the etiology of one disease is obscure.

Disease associations may be more apparent than real. Two diseases may produce similar signs, symptoms, or laboratory findings, thus leading to a greater chance of *diagnosis* of one disease if the other is present. Also, diseases are detected in the clinic, hospital, or at autopsy, and the presence of more than one disease may make it more likely for a person to show up at one of these diagnostic facilities. Due to this and other selective factors, diseases may appear to be associated at a medical facility even when they are not associated in the general population. Further discussion of disease associations and the potential fallacies involved may be found in Berkson (1946), Mainland (1953), Wijsman (1958), and Friedman (1968).

Even false associations due to selection may be useful to the clinician. For example, an association between inguinal hernia and colon cancer has been noted on the surgical ward (Terezis et al., 1963). Even if this association is not present in the general population, it still may be wise for surgeons to look for colon cancer in their patients with hernias.

REFERENCES

Berkson, J. 1946. Limitations of the application of fourfold table analysis to hospital data. *Biometrics Bull.*, **2**:47–53.

Bross, I. D. J. 1966. Spurious effects from an extraneous variable. *J. Chronic Dis.*, **19**:637–647.

Friedman, G. D. 1967. Cigarette smoking and geographic variation in coronary heart disease mortality in the United States. *J. Chron. Dis.*, **20**:769–779.

Friedman, G. D. 1968. The relationship between coronary heart disease and gallbladder disease: A critical review. *Ann. Intern. Med.*, **68**:222–235.

Friedman, G. D., A. B. Siegelaub, C. C. Seltzer, R. Feldman, and M. F. Collen. 1973. Smoking habits and the leukocyte count. *Arch. Environ. Health*, **26**:137–143.

Hill, A. B., *Principles of Medical Statistics*, 9th edition. (London: Oxford University Press, 1971).

Ipsen, J., and P. Feigl, *Bancroft's Introduction to Biostatistics.* (New York: Harper and Row, 1970).

Larsen, P. S., and H. Silvette, *Tobacco: Experimental and Clinical Studies* Supplement I. (Baltimore: Williams and Wilkins, 1968), pp. 346–362.

MacMahon, B., and T. F. Pugh, *Epidemiology: Principles and Methods.* (Boston: Little, Brown, 1970).

Mainland, D. 1953. The risk of fallacious conclusions from autopsy data of the incidence of diseases with applications to heart disease. *Am. Heart J.*, **45**:644–654.

Morrison, D. F., *Multivariate Statistical Methods.* (New York: McGraw-Hill Book Company, 1967).

Robinson, W. S. 1950. Ecological correlations and the behavior of individuals. *Am. Sociol. Rev.*, **15**:351–357.

Susser, M., *Causal Thinking in the Health Sciences: Concepts and Strategies of Epidemiology.* (New York: Oxford University Press, 1973).

Terezis, L. N., W. C. Davis, and F. C. Jackson. 1963. Carcinoma of the colon associated with inguinal hernia. *New Engl. J. Med.*, **268**:774.

Truett, J., J. Cornfield, and W. Kannel. 1967. A multivariate analysis of the risk of coronary heart disease in Framingham. *J. Chron. Dis.*, **20**:511–524.

Vessey, M. P., and R. Doll. 1968. Investigation of relation between use of oral contraceptives and thromboembolic disease. *Brit. Med. J.*, **2**:199–205.

Wijsman, R. A. 1958. Contribution to the study of the question of associations between two diseases. *Human Biology*, **30**:219–236.

Yerushalmy, J., Statistical considerations and evaluation of epidemiological evidence, in *Tobacco and Health* edited by G. James and T. Rosenthal. (Springfield, Ill.: Charles C Thomas, 1962), pp. 208–230.

Chapter 12

How to Carry Out a Study

Many health-care professionals wish to conduct a modest clinical or epidemiologic study. Hoping to answer one or more interesting questions, they find themselves in a good position to collect and analyze some appropriate data. However, to someone without previous research experience, the task often appears awesome, and it is not at all clear how to proceed.

This chapter is written as a general guide for the novice who wishes to carry out such a study. Obviously, each research project and each study setting presents unique problems which cannot be dealt with here. What will be presented is a general approach which emphasizes the practical difficulties that are frequently troublesome to the beginner.

Defining the Problem

The first step—and one of the most difficult ones—is defining the problem and choosing the question or questions to be answered.

There is a tendency for the novice at research to ask questions that are diffuse or vague. Instead, the problem must be stated in terms of clear, simple, answerable questions.

An example of a vague unachievable goal for a specific study would be *to elucidate the role of psychological factors in coronary heart disease.* It is not clear whether the "role . . . in coronary heart disease" refers to causation of the disease, outcome of disease, the patient's attitude toward the disease, or something entirely different. Furthermore, both "coronary heart disease" and "psychological factors" are very broad terms. Better, because they are clear and answerable, are specific aims or questions such as, *Determine the proportion of patients with myocardial infarction who develop severe emotional depression during hospitalization. Do attacks of angina pectoris occur more frequently during periods when patients are anxious?* Or, *Is there an increased risk of sudden cardiac death within a year after the death of a spouse?*

Intimately involved in the asking of vague, overly broad questions is the tendency to be too ambitious. The new researcher wishes to make important discoveries and solve big problems. These unrealistic expectations can only lead to failure and disappointment. For the most part, medical science progresses gradually by very small steps. So much of health care is based on tenuous evidence and incomplete knowledge that a careful study of a simple question will be a worthwhile contribution, of which any scientist should be proud.

Reviewing the Relevant Literature

Once a problem has been selected, the scientific papers describing previous related work should be read carefully. In addition to learning what is already known about the question, the investigator will become familiar with problems that others have faced, using various study methods. One should be especially alert for related variables which can be measured or controlled in the planned study so that embarrassing spurious correlations can be recognized or avoided. For example, no investigation of a possible etiologic factor in lung cancer would be respectable if smoking habits were not measured or taken into account.

The usual result of a literature review will be a realization of how *little* is known about the particular topic one wishes to investigate. Seemingly authoritative statements and accepted medical doctrines, perpetuated through textbooks and lectures, often turn out to be supported by the most meager of evidence, if any can be found at all! For example, my own experience in reviewing the literature for an epidemiologic study of gallbladder disease was an inability to find any evidence for the "fair" and "forty" parts of the doctrine that persons who are "fair, fat, and forty" are especially prone to gallstones. Indeed, the study did not confirm these traits as predisposing factors.

Many other examples could be mentioned of beliefs that are based on little or no evidence or on the results of poorly conducted studies. In these instances, a literature review will provide encouragement for proceeding with the proposed study. On the other hand, if it is evident that the question has already been well answered, a related problem may come to mind—one that can be studied just as well.

Preparing a Protocol

The next essential step is the preparation of a study protocol. Even though the beginning investigator may feel that he has clearly in mind what he plans to do, it is extremely important to set down the plan in writing.

A written protocol serves three major purposes. First of all, when one writes the protocol, ideas and procedures must be clearly defined and spelled out. Usually the plan in one's mind is not as clear and logical as was hoped, and the gaps and flaws are easier to recognize and correct when the plan is seen on paper. Secondly, a written protocol can be studied by anyone whose advice is desired or whose approval is required. Thirdly, any person working to carry out the study, even the investigator himself, may forget some method or procedure to be followed. The written protocol constitutes a permanent record that can be referred to, so that methods do not change unnecessarily during the conduct of the study.

Some persons have such an abhorrence of writing that the preparation of a protocol is an almost insurmountable obstacle to carrying out a study. If so, it is probably better just to quit at this point, since even if some data are collected and analyzed, the results will probably never be written up and no one else can adequately study the findings. Another alternative for a nonwriter with a good idea for a research project is to team up with a co-investigator who is willing and able to write the protocol and the final report.

Contents of the protocol Research grant applications may require strict adherence to prescribed contents arranged in a particular order. For example, a recent communication from the U.S. National Institutes of Health listed the following required elements for a grant application.

Broad statement of objectives
Detailed budget for the first year
Budget estimates for subsequent years
Biographical sketches for all professional personnel
Research Plan

  A Introduction
    1 Overall objective or long-term goal
    2 Background: significant previous work and current status of research
    3 Rationale behind the proposed approach to the problem
  B Specific aims
  C Methods of procedure—methods used, data to be collected, how the data will be analyzed and interpreted, possible pitfalls and limitations, tentative schedule
  D Significance of the proposed work
  E Facilities available
  F Collaborative arrangements, if any
  G Appendix—various detailed descriptions, letters confirming proposed collaboration, etc.

A protocol prepared for local use may be shorter and simpler but should contain at least the following elements, unless there is good reason for omitting any.

1 A brief statement of the specific question(s) to be answered and/or the specific aim(s) of the study

2 Background and significance of the study. This should be a pertinent nonrambling discussion of what is known and not known about the problem and why the proposed study is worthwhile or important.

3 Methods. Included should be a description of the study subjects—how they are to be selected and how many there are likely to be. The data to be collected and the methods for collecting them should be described. Uniform criteria for diagnosis of disease and for decisions as to the presence or absence of a characteristic or outcome should be listed. Data analysis methods should also be presented, preferably with some sample blank tables showing how the data will be organized. Plans for safeguarding the rights and welfare of the subjects and the method of obtaining their informed consent (if needed) should be explained.

4 An approximate time schedule for carrying out the various aspects of the study.

5 A budget, if financial support is being requested, with explanation of any personnel and other costs whose requirement is not obvious.

Consultation

After a draft of the protocol has been written, it is wise to seek some expert consultation before proceeding any further. Many potential problems and difficulties will be quickly spotted by knowledgeable persons reviewing the protocol and discussing the proposed research.

It should be no reflection on one's intelligence and skill to ask for advice. No one can foresee all the problems that may develop in his own study. A consultant will respect the investigator who draws up a protocol as well as he can and then admits that he is fallible.

Help can come from persons in a number of disciplines. An experienced investigator who has worked in the area to be studied can perhaps provide the most comprehensive view of the problem. A clinician who specializes in the area of study will often provide some fresh insights into the subject matter derived from experience with patients and from familiarity with the current literature. Epidemiologists and, particularly, biostatisticians are professionally concerned with study design and data analysis and can provide guidance on these aspects of the study. The choice of appropriate statistical tests and the determination of whether or not the proposed sample size is adequate to obtain meaningful information, are of particular concern to the biostatistician.

The protocol should now be revised taking into account the suggestions of the consultants.

Presenting the Study Plan to Other Key Individuals

At this time the investigator should inform all the responsible persons whose approval or cooperation is either required or desirable. Proposed research in medical or academic institutions should be presented to appropriate departmental heads and/or hospital administrators. Often there will be a committee specially designated to review and approve of studies. Epidemiologic studies in the community should be described to local health officials and to the medical society.

In addition to gaining the required approvals, the investigator may receive valuable practical suggestions and other assistance from these individuals, such as introductions to physicians who may permit the study of their own patients. The investigator may also learn of other similar or related research that is under way. Cooperation with other investigators may help avoid duplication of effort and may lead to sharing of resources and, possibly, even of data.

Data Collection Methods

The data to be collected—whether by observation or interview of subjects, by chart review, laboratory tests, or however—must be recorded in a systematic and orderly manner. The usual method of bringing order into the data-recording process is by the use of standard forms. Careful attention to preparation of a form, even if only a few items need to be recorded on it, will save the investigator from much trouble and grief later on.

One or more forms will be used for each study subject. Each form should provide space for identification of the subject and for recording the necessary data about him.

If mechanical or electronic data processors are to be used for analysis, the format for recording data on the form should meet the requirements of these devices. Each unit of information must be recorded in a particular space on each form. Each space is ordinarily assigned a column number to correspond with the column on a punch card to which that unit of information will be transferred. Currently, most data processing equipment accepts information from 80-column punch cards, but because of local variations, the investigator should seek advice from data processing personnel at his institution before drawing up the form.

For recording quantitative information, specific spaces or boxes should be designated so that the same digit (e.g., the "ones," "tens," or "hundreds" digit) is entered into the same space on each form, and the location of the decimal point is uniform. If the value to be recorded is relatively small and does not require all the assigned spaces, zeros should be written in the spaces to the left, which would not otherwise be filled in. Adequate spaces should be provided for all possible values of any particular measurement and for recording that the value is unknown. Special instructions for recording each measurement may be located on the form itself or in an accompanying manual.

For example, suppose an investigator wishes to record the serum-glucose level at admission to the hospital and he provides three spaces on his form, to be transferred, say, to columns 20–22 of the punch card, as follows:

Serum glucose (mg/100 ml)   ☐☐☐

                                              Cols. 20–22

At first glance this may seem adequate, but consider what might go wrong if a research assistant tries to use these spaces for three patients, one with a value of 72, one with 1,021, and one for whom the test was not done. Without special instructions to use the two boxes on the right for two-digit numbers, the value of 72 might be recorded as ⎡7⎤⎡2⎤⎡ ⎤, which will be treated by the computer or card sorter as 720. In recording the value 1,021 the naïve research assistant might well write 1 ⎡0⎤⎡2⎤⎡1⎤ not realizing that what is outside the three boxes will be lost in data processing. The investigator should have anticipated the possibility of the occasional extremely high value for a patient suffering from diabetic acidosis and provided four boxes instead of three. If there is good reason to limit the spaces to three, another less-satisfactory alternative is to make a rule for high values such as "Code 999 for values of 999 or greater. Write actual value below." The value can then be referred to if needed. However, the computer will not be able to compute an accurate mean if 999 is always substituted for greater values.

For the patient with no glucose determination the research assistant may leave the space blank. But 6 months later when the data are to be analyzed, and the research assistant has moved to another city, the investigator will not be sure whether the blank spaces represent an unknown value or whether the assistant forgot to fill in the spaces. It is better to indicate "test not done" with a particular number that could not represent a possible value of the variable. Consideration of these potential problems leads to the improved version of the portion of the form for recording serum glucose as follows:

Serum glucose (mg/100 ml)   ☐☐☐☐
                                                  Cols. 20–23

(Record one-, two-, and three-digit numbers
as far to the right as possible, and
fill in the left boxes with zeros.
If test not done, record 9999)

Qualitative data, such as diagnostic categories, or "yes" or "no" responses, usually require the assignment of code numbers to each response if data processing devices are to be used. Consider marital status, for example. Without coding, a data collection form might show marital status as follows:

Marital status (check appropriate category)

☐ Single   ☐ Widowed
☐ Married   ☐ Divorced
☐ Separated   ☐ Unknown

The responses could be coded into a single digit if a number were assigned to each category. The digit could be recorded in a space or box on the same sheet or onto a separate code sheet. For example, note how marital status can be coded into one digit to be transferred to, say, Col. 17 on a punch card.

Marital status (enter appropriate number into box)   ☐

1	Single	**4**	Widowed	Col. 17
2	Married	**5**	Divorced	
3	Separated	**6**	Unknown	

Precoded forms permit the correct category to be marked and coded automatically. For example:

Marital status (circle number next to appropriate category)

Single	1	⎫
Married	2	⎪
Separated	3	⎬ Col. 17
Widowed	4	⎪
Divorced	5	⎪
Unknown	6	⎭

There are advantages and disadvantages to each type of form. Some general principles to consider are:

The less rewriting or transcribing of data that is needed, the less chance for error.

The less complex the form, the less chance for error.

Most physicians and other professionals neither like to code nor do a good job of coding. If such individuals are to record data, it is often necessary to design a form they will use, and pay someone else to do the coding.

In preparing to record qualitative data, a category should be provided for every possibility except the very rare ones. Writing of additional information on the form in longhand should be kept at a minimum because this sort of information is difficult to analyze and relate to the other variables. Consider, for example, a study of factors related to adverse reactions to anticoagulant drugs. One item of information that will be desired about each patient is the medical condition for which the anticoagulant is given. The investigator could set up his code sheet as follows:

Condition for which anticoagulant was given:_____
_____
_____

However, he might later find it difficult to summarize these data and combine patients into categories. Using his clinical experience to anticipate the possibilities, he would find the data easier to analyze and present by providing several mutually exclusive categories, as follows:

Condition for which anticoagulant was given: ☐☐
01 Pulmonary embolism   Cols. 32–33
02 Thrombophlebitis
03 Pulmonary embolism and thrombophlebitis
04 Myocardial infarction
05 Myocardial infarction with mural thrombosis and peripheral embolism
06 Rheumatic heart disease
07 Rheumatic heart disease with peripheral embolism
08 Atrial fibrillation or flutter
09 Atrial fibrillation or flutter with peripheral embolism
10 Atrial fibrillation or flutter with therapeutic conversion
11 Prosthetic heart valve
12 Transient cerebral ischemic attacks
13 Other cerebrovascular disease, specify _____
14 Other disease, specify _____
15 Combinations of above, specify _____
_____

Note the last three categories which involve some specification in longhand. These permit the recording of unanticipated conditions. But provision of the other common categories will reduce the need for longhand recording to a very small fraction of the cases.

When specifying categories for data-collection forms it is wise to avoid making these categories too broad. Overly broad categories lead to the loss of valuable information. For example, categories, 08,

09, and 10 above, might have been combined under a more inclusive category "atrial fibrillation or flutter," but then, important clinical distinctions among these cases could not be made without referring to the chart again. Frequently the investigator assumes that broad categories will be adequate for the needs of the study. Later on when the data are analyzed, unanticipated questions arise which could have been answered if narrower categories had been used.

Broad categories may prove especially troublesome when quantitative variables are recorded. In providing for the coding of serum glucose it might initially seem reasonable to have only 7 categories:

1 Less than 50 mg/100 ml
2 50–99
3 100–199
4 200–499
5 500–999
6 1,000+
7 Test not done

With luck, this might be perfectly adequate. However, if another investigator's study shows an important difference in findings between persons whose glucose level is less than 350 mg/100 ml and those whose glucose is 350 mg/100 ml or greater, the broad categories chosen will not permit data analysis to determine whether the breakpoint at 350 mg/100 ml can be confirmed. Furthermore, it is not possible to compute accurate means and standard deviations with the crude breakdown as shown above.

Thus it is best to record quantitative values exactly as they come from the measuring device. This allows for maximum flexibility and permits the investigator subsequently to use any grouping he desires.

Pretesting of Data Collection

No matter how carefully the data collection is planned, problems will come to light after starting. That is why it is important to pretest procedures and forms before the study formally begins.

Suppose, for example, that data for a study of cardiovascular disease are to be collected in a mobile facility in which volunteer subjects are scheduled to pass from station to station every 5 minutes for a series of procedures. It may turn out that the electrocardiogram takes 8 minutes, on the average, instead of the planned 5 minutes. As a result subjects may pile up at earlier stations if there was no provision for a waiting area in case of delays. It may therefore be necessary to slow down the examination schedule, or provide two electrocardiographic stations, or set up a waiting area. This problem should be uncovered and solved during pretesting. If not, and the subjects have to wait or get the impression that the study is disorganized, cooperation may be seriously impaired.

Similarly, a series of interview questions may seem perfectly clear and appropriate when they are written down. Yet when study subjects are actually asked these questions they may not understand, or be offended, or give responses that were not anticipated. In a study of radiation exposure, for example, the investigator may consider it perfectly reasonable to ask, "Have you ever received x-ray or isotope therapy?" It will undoubtedly turn out that some subjects answer "yes" because they misinterpret the question to mean x-ray examinations. The question will have to be reworded and supplemented with additional clarifying questions in case of a "yes" response. Problems such as these quickly become apparent when an interview is tried out on friends and associates first, and then on some persons similar to the potential study subjects, but not officially part of the study.

Even abstracting data from charts requires pretesting. It seems perfectly reasonable to ask a research assistant reviewing hospital charts to record the patients' blood pressure at the time of admission. When the assistant looks at the first few charts it will be noted that some, but not all, patients are admitted to a ward from the emergency room, where the blood pressure was recorded by the intern. There is also a blood pressure recorded as the first of a series of blood pressures on the nurse's vital signs chart. In addition, the intern and resident on the ward each performed an initial physical examination in which the blood pressure was recorded. It is apparent that some rule will be required for selecting the blood pressure to be used, if any consistency is to be achieved. Review of a few charts will also reveal that one of the interns has recorded two diastolic pressures, one at the muffling and one at the disappearance of Korotkov's sounds. Thus another decision is required—which one to use.

To mention other examples, the investigator may ask a chart reviewer to indicate whether the patient has a history of hypertension—yes or no. The chart reviewer will find, for a particular patient, that one physician records such a history and another does not. Which physician's history should be used? Or, on a previous hospitalization one blood pressure of 150/105 was recorded. Does this constitute a history of hypertension? Again, decisions and further clarification are needed. Or, the form was constructed so as to provide spaces for three digits for recording systolic pressure and two for diastolic, because it was forgotten that the diastolic is frequently greater than 99 mm Hg. Pretesting will reveal the need to change the form.

Data Collection

If the investigator is relying on others to collect and record the data, he should supervise this aspect of the study closely, especially during the early stages. The work of persons collecting the data should be observed, and completed data collection forms should be checked carefully. In this way, the investigator can ensure that his study plan is being followed.

Not all problems will have been discovered during pretesting. Further changes in procedures and forms may have to be made after the study officially begins. These modifications should be kept to a minimum in order to avoid inconsistencies in the data. Any changes or new rules to be followed should be recorded as additions to the protocol.

Data Analysis

Data analysis for most epidemiologic or clinical-outcome studies mainly involves sorting into categories and counting, then computing proportions, rates, means, and other group characteristics.

In order to proceed in an orderly fashion and end up with the answers that were desired in the first place, it is often helpful to draw up some blank tables showing the format for displaying the results of data analysis as they would be presented in a final report. These tables are then filled in with the appropriate counts, rates, and so on when these results become available.

For the novice, preparing blank tables is often quite difficult, requiring a good deal of patience and self-discipline. However, the results are well worth the effort and, with experience, subsequent table-making becomes much easier.

Data analysis tables should show the results broken down by age, sex, and other pertinent variables. In addition to showing the key results that one is after, they should show the numbers upon which these results are based. For example, Table 12-1, below, showing just incidence rates, is inadequate. The counts upon which these rates are based, should also be listed, as in Table 12-2.

Table 12-1   Incomplete Table Showing Only Incidence Rates by Age and Sex (Fictitious Data)

Age	Annual incidence rate/1,000
Men	
20–29	16.5
30–39	22.8
40–49	23.4
50–59	42.4
60–69	77.1
Total	33.3
Women	
20–29	5.5
30–39	8.6
40–49	10.5
50–59	20.9
60–69	40.6
Total	16.2

Table 12-2 Complete Table Showing Incidence Rates by Age and Sex and the Numbers upon Which They Are Based (Fictitious Data)

Age	Population at risk	Number of new cases during the year	Annual incidence rate/1,000
Men			
20–29	1,572	26	16.5
30–39	1,494	34	22.8
40–49	2,012	47	23.4
50–59	1,629	69	42.4
60–69	1,077	83	77.1
Total	7,784	259	33.3
Women			
20–29	1,827	10	5.5
30–39	2,203	19	8.6
40–49	2,570	27	10.5
50–59	1,912	40	20.9
60–69	1,698	69	40.6
Total	10,210	165	16.2

Similarly, when means and standard deviations are shown, the number of persons entering into each of these computations should be given.

The actual work of data processing can be carried out in a variety of ways. The proper choice of method depends on how many subjects are involved and the complexity of the analysis. If only a few counts and proportions are to be determined for a few dozen subjects, manual counting of items on the data collection forms will be quite adequate. With increasing numbers and tabulations, the investigator may wish to sort and count his data using special cards, available at stationery stores, with holes punched near the edges. Each subject's data are recorded on one of these cards. The presence of a particular characteristic can be shown on the card by punching away the thin strip of cardboard that separates the hole from the edge. When the cards are lined up behind each other, a long needle is passed through the corresponding hole in all cards and then lifted. The cards representing persons with the particular characteristic will drop away from the rest.

Even more helpful, and useful for studies with hundreds or even thousands of subjects, is the electric card-sorting machine. Data are keypunched onto special cards (most often with 80 columns, one for each digit). These cards are rapidly sorted by the machine into subgroups, and the number of cards in each subgroup is counted at the same time. Card sorters of this type are widely available, and the investigator can easily learn to operate one in a few minutes.

After any of the above sorting and counting methods are used, the arithmetic necessary for computing rates, means, statistical-significance tests, and so on, may be conveniently done on an electric desk calculator.

If a great number of counts and sorts have to be done on large numbers of subjects and/or if complex mathematical calculations are required, then the electronic digital computer is the ideal data-analysis tool. Voluminous data may be transferred from punch cards to a reel of magnetic tape, which may be used repeatedly for as many analyses as are desired. To use a computer, the investigator must usually obtain the services of a programmer or else learn to program it himself. If a programmer is employed, the investigator will have to explain in meticulous detail exactly what he wants. Various systems are being developed to make it easier for an investigator with little knowledge of programming to communicate directly with the computer.

Preparing the Final Report

The difficult job of preparing the scientific paper describing the study becomes a much less imposing task if the investigator writes portions of it during the course of the investigation.

The introductory section of the paper briefly outlines the problem and the purpose of the study. Note that this material has already been set down in preparing the written protocol. All that has to be done is to make any modifications that seem necessary for a final paper, or that come to mind now that data collection and analysis are completed.

Similarly, the Methods section of the paper can be readily

adapted from the protocol. It should describe exactly what was done and, in addition, inform the reader how subjects were selected for study, how many were included or excluded and the reasons for exclusion. Criteria for classifying subjects and for decisions as to outcomes should be spelled out.

Writing the Results and Discussion sections is simplified if the investigator takes advantage of the fact that the results usually appear in stages. Tables of data are usually completed one at a time. As the investigator prepares or receives each table, he should immediately write a paragraph or two describing it for the Results section and a paragraph or two discussing the implication of this result for the Discussion section. Then, by the time the data are completely analyzed, most of the writing will be done. The Results and Discussion will still have to be organized and edited, but the task of writing it will not have to be faced all at once.

In the Discussion section the implications of the study and its relation to previous work should be described. In addition, the difficulties, problems, and potential errors and biases of the present investigation should be reviewed. All investigations have some obvious limitations and others that are not so obvious. It is best if the investigator recognizes and points these out himself, before someone else does.

Importance of Good Communication

Science is a *social* process. Each investigation is related to previous work, either attempting to confirm it or, usually, to build upon it. Investigators need to know and understand what others have done and are doing. It is, therefore, an important responsibility to present a study as fully and clearly as possible.

A paper, or an oral presentation at a meeting, should be clear and simple. Jargon and unnecessarily complex or obscure terminology should be avoided. Although tables of data in a written paper should be complete, they need not be repetitious. Thus, after the basic numbers have been shown once (as in Table 12-2), they do not have to be repeated over and over again. Some relationships may be communicated most clearly by means of graphs and figures; these visual aids should be used freely.

In preparing slides or charts to accompany an oral presentation, the temptation to crowd a lot of information into one slide should be resisted. Each slide should have only a few lines or numbers, displayed with large characters, easily seen by those in the back of the room.

Importance of Investigator Worry

Many things can go wrong and many errors can occur during a study. Therefore it is essential that, preferably, the investigator himself, or else a conscientious person responsible to the investigator, *worry about details*. The careful investigator might well adopt a questioning or even a suspicious attitude toward his study.

In addition to observing the process of data collection, as recommended above, the investigator should see to it that every data-recording form is checked carefully by someone other than the person who filled it out, to detect and correct omissions and obvious errors. Copies should be made of all completed data collection forms so that the original information will still be available if any forms are lost. Complete lists and counts of all study subjects should be maintained to provide a check against lost forms. It is surprising how often forms become misplaced or piles of punch cards fall behind a desk. Keypunching of data should be verified, which involves repeating the keypunching on a machine that detects discrepancies.

All mathematical calculations should be done twice by two different persons. The investigator should be sure to have his own work double-checked by a conscientious individual. Computer programs should be tested on small samples of data and the results compared with hand calculations.

Data tables should be checked to make sure that all the numbers are correct and add up to the totals shown. Surprising or inconsistent results should provoke redoubled efforts to check whether something has gone wrong.

Finally, it would be sad, indeed, if after all this work the resulting paper were to contain misleading typographical or printing errors. The manuscript and galley proofs should be proofread carefully.

Chapter 13

Epidemiology and Patient Care

Epidemiology is quite important in patient care. Clinical decisions are greatly affected by knowledge of the patterns of disease occurrence in populations. Some of the ways that diagnosis and treatment are, or should be, related to epidemiologic knowledge and principles will be discussed in this chapter.

Epidemiology and Diagnosis

In making a diagnosis, the physician must select from the hundreds of known diseases that one which most probably fits the patient's clinical picture. In assessing the probability of a given condition being present, the physician is strongly influenced by an awareness of what diseases are prevalent in his community at the time. During an influenza epidemic, for example, a patient exhibiting fever, headache, weakness, and myalgia would be promptly diagnosed as having influenza; whereas, with no such epidemic taking place,

laboratory tests would probably be ordered to rule out other explanations for the illness. Similarly, in the United States in the 1970's,
if a patient presents with congestive heart failure, diphtheritic or
Chagas' myocarditis need rarely be considered.

Descriptive epidemiologic findings indicating subgroups of the
population in which a disease has a low or high prevalence are also
useful for diagnosis. Knowing that a patient is of a particular age or
sex or occupation, or that he comes from a certain part of the
country, is very helpful in narrowing down the probable diseases he
or she might have. For example, if a patient has lived in the San
Joaquin Valley of California, coccidioidomycosis should be strongly
suspected as the disease responsible for a nonspecific lung lesion
seen on his chest x-ray.

The use of epidemiologic knowledge in the diagnosis of heart
disease was well described by Dry (1943) who quoted "a cardiologist
of long experience" as follows:

> When I am called to see a patient with heart disease that is not
> of almost self-evident nature I find out certain things before I
> enter the room. I know whether the patient is a baby, a child, an
> adolescent, or an adult. If he is an adult, I find out in what age
> range he falls. There are certain heart diseases found com-
> monly in certain ages and rarely found in persons of other ages.
> I have made my first step in probable diagnosis right then.
>
> Then, particularly if the patient is an adult, I must know
> whether he is male or female, for there is a sex predilection for
> certain diseases of the heart. That's my second step and I have
> narrowed the probable diagnosis down further.
>
> Next, I find out from the history what he has been exposed
> to. What diseases has he had? What kind of life has he lived?
> Has he suffered important hardships, been a rounder? Is he or
> she a successful, hard driving person? How much does he eat,
> smoke and drink? In what condition is his general health? Such
> questions as these narrow the problem down further. I am pretty
> well along in logical diagnosis by exclusion before I cross the
> threshold.
>
> Then I do cross it but I'm in no hurry. I shake hands with the
> patient, feel his pulse. I get certain impressions that way. I
> look at him, talk to him and size him up as a man and a doctor
> rather than as a cardiologist. I ask him questions about his

specific complaints and continue to ply him with questions until I have the picture in my own mind of just what he has been experiencing subjectively. It is not enough to know, for instance, that he has pain in his chest or shortness of breath because either may indicate serious heart disease or a condition that is relatively innocent. Thus I have secured further background and some of what already was in my mind when I was standing in the hall has been either reinforced or refuted.

Then I put my hands and my stethoscope on his chest in the course of a complete and thorough examination. Next I review the x-ray and the electrocardiogram. I ought to get every bit of evidence I can, but I honestly doubt if any of it is usually as important as the thinking I did in the hall and at the bedside before I touched the patient or had any apparatus applied to him.

Analytic Studies to Improve Methods of Diagnosis

Population studies, quite analogous to analytic epidemiologic studies, have been used to refine diagnostic methods. Just as epidemiology traditionally studies the associations between a disease and etiologic or predictive factors, the same approach may be used to study the associations between a disease and symptoms, signs, or laboratory tests. These, after all, constitute the information that is used to make a diagnosis.

Because of the current popularity of laboratory tests, one need only glance through a volume of issues of any leading medical journal to find examples of studies showing how a particular test may be used to help distinguish between persons with and without a particular disease, or between different categories of patients with the same disease. Ordinarily, the test will be performed on different patient groups, plus some "normal controls." The distributions of the test results in each of these groups are then compared. When any two distributions appear quite different and show little overlap, the test is valuable in discriminating between the two groups; that is, the test is helpful in determining whether a patient belongs to one group or the other.

The value of a symptom in distinguishing between persons with and without a disease may be investigated similarly. Two recent population studies are examples of great interest because they showed that certain traditional clinical teachings about the relationship between a disease and a symptom are probably incorrect.

One of these studies (Price, 1963) looked closely at the relationship between various types of indigestion or dyspepsia and gallbladder disease. It had long been taught by some authorities that chronic epigastric pain, flatulence, heartburn, and intolerance to fatty and other types of foods could often be due to a diseased gallbladder. A total of 204 women, ages 50–70, were identified in one urban general-practice patient roster in the United Kingdom. Of these women, 142, or 70 percent, agreed to be interviewed concerning these symptoms. Each patient later had an x-ray of the gallbladder, by means of which 24 were shown to have gallstones or a poorly functioning gallbladder.

The relative frequency of fatty-food intolerance and of each of the other "typical" symptoms was quite similar in the groups with normal and abnormal gallbladders. Altogether, dyspepsia was quite a common symptom, afflicting about half of each group. The type of indigestion experienced by the abnormal group did not differ appreciably from that reported by normals. The author concluded that among women, ages 50–70, the presence of both gallbladder disease and dyspepsia is coincidental, and that these symptoms can not assist in the diagnosis of gallbladder disease and should not influence its treatment.

In another study of this type, Weiss (1972) analyzed data from the 1960–1962 U.S. National Health Survey to explore the relationship between hypertension and certain symptoms, long regarded as being due to this condition. Responses to questions about these symptoms on a self-administered questionnaire were studied in relation to blood pressure subsequently measured by a physician. Headache, epistaxis, and tinnitus showed no relationship to either systolic or diastolic pressure. A history of dizziness was more prevalent only in those hypertensives with a very high diastolic pressure. Fainting was inversely related to blood pressure, being reported more frequently by those with lower pressures.

It is not surprising that many physicians have accepted the teaching that gallbladder disease produces fatty-food intolerance and hypertension produces headache. First of all, these relationships, particularly the former, can be "explained" physiologically. Secondly, these symptoms are quite common; thus it is not surprising to find patients complaining of them. Nevertheless, by examining these symptom-disease relationships in general population groups, the epidemiologic approach can put them in proper perspective.

"Normal" Values

Returning again to laboratory tests and other quantitative measurements, practicing physicians and laboratory directors are in the habit of dividing the distributions of these findings into two parts, the "normal" and the "abnormal." Having a clear dividing line or "normal limit" between the two alternatives makes it easier to make decisions. If the patient is normal, he can be reassured; if he or she is abnormal, some action must be taken. Thus, it is important to understand how normal limits are arrived at.

Unfortunately, much confusion surrounds this area because the term "normal" has more than one meaning. As used above it means "good" or "desirable" or "healthy." Another important meaning is "usual" or "frequent." In this sense, it is normal for an older person to have gray hair. This says that the occurrence is common but implies nothing either way about desirability. As if these two definitions did not cause sufficient confusion, there is a third meaning having to do with the shape of a distribution curve that is often observed in studies of human characteristics. This symmetrical, bell-shaped curve is referred to as the "Gaussian" or "normal" distribution curve.

One method that has been used to define the "normal-healthy" has been to determine the "normal-usual." That is, the particular test is applied to a large population. A cutoff point is applied to one or both ends of the distribution curve so that an arbitrary small percentage, say 5 percent or 1 percent of the population, will be called abnormal. Clearly, by this method, the normal range is merely the usual range; but it is easy to drift into the view that normal-usual means normal-healthy.

This method for determining normal-healthy limits can be improved upon by finding the normal-usual values in a population that is known to be healthy. Unfortunately, the healthy group studied is often small and select—for example, a group of medical or nursing students. Thus it is hard to be sure whether test values associated with health in these groups would also be associated with health in persons of different ages and circumstances.

Even better than studying a healthy group alone is to determine the test values in two groups, one that is healthy and one which has the disease being tested for. The result will usually be two overlapping distributions as shown in Fig. 13-1. Outside the area where the distributions overlap, a test result clearly identifies the presence or absence of disease. If a patient's value falls into the area of overlap, he has a chance of belonging to either the normal or abnormal group. Choosing one cutoff point will thus result in errors in classification; that is, there will be some truly normal individuals on the abnormal side of the cutoff point who will, therefore, be called abnormal, and there will be some truly abnormal individuals who will be considered normal.

These two types of classification errors can be expressed quantitatively in terms of the *sensitivity* and the *specificity* of a test. Sensitivity is the proportion of truly diseased who are called diseased by the test. Specificity is the proportion of truly nondiseased persons who are so identified by the test. In the example shown in Fig. 13-1 it is apparent that these two measures are inversely related to one another. Shifting the cutoff point to the left will increase sensitivity at the cost of specificity. That is, a higher percentage of sick persons will be called sick but a smaller percentage of the well will be called well. Moving the cutoff point to the right will increase specificity while decreasing sensitivity. More of the well will be called well but less sickness will be detected.

In setting the normal cutoff point, then, attention must be paid to the purpose of the test. If it is very important not to miss a particular disease which is both treatable and serious, one usually favors sensitivity over specificity, hoping to correctly identify as many cases as possible. On the other hand, if detecting a disease results in little benefit while falsely labeling normal persons as sick results in much worry and cost, specificity is to be preferred.

Unfortunately, the physician's desire for a nice cutoff point has been dealt a rather serious blow by recent epidemiologic studies, particularly in cardiovascular disease. For important coronary risk

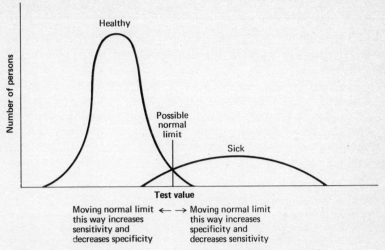

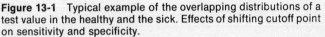

Moving normal limit ← — → Moving normal limit
this way increases   this way increases
sensitivity and   specificity and
decreases specificity   decreases sensitivity

Figure 13-1 Typical example of the overlapping distributions of a test value in the healthy and the sick. Effects of shifting cutoff point on sensitivity and specificity.

factors such as blood pressure and cholesterol, it appears that within the range usually observed in this country there is no cutoff point between a safe and unsafe level. That is, the lower the level, the better off one is. There is no single level above which treatment should be given. Decisions to treat an elevated coronary risk factor must be based not only on the level of the risk factor itself but on the presence or absence of other indicators of risk. Thus, one is more apt to try to lower a serum-cholesterol level of 260 mg/100 ml if it is found in a middle-aged man who also smokes cigarettes and has a blood pressure of 150/95.

Serum cholesterol provides an excellent demonstration of the distinction between normal-usual and normal-healthy. It is not at all unusual to find a middle-aged man with a serum-cholesterol level which should hardly be considered as indicative of good health, even if the man feels well. Specifically, there is abundant epidemiologic evidence that *one-fourth* of men, i.e., those who happen to belong to the highest quartile of the cholesterol distribution, have three to four times the risk of developing clinical coronary heart disease as men in the lowest quartile. Knowing that about one in every five men in this highest quartile will develop clinical coronary heart disease in the next 10 years hardly leads to confidence that they are normal-healthy, especially since there is mounting evidence that medical attention to their diet and living habits may reduce their high risk.

Epidemiologic studies have shown that many characteristics that have been regarded as normal because they are usual in persons who presently feel well are associated with a high probability of *future* disease. A preventive approach implies that these characteristics can no longer be regarded as consistent with good health.

Practicing Preventive Medicine in the Office or Clinic

Epidemiologic knowledge fosters the practice of preventive medicine in the medical office. Knowledge of the factors and characteristics which *cause* or *predict* the development of a disease permits identifying individuals who are at high risk of developing it. It may then be possible to prescribe measures for these patients that will prevent or at least delay the onset of the disease.

Nowadays, pediatricians are quite comfortable with the office practice of preventive medicine. Immunizations and well-baby care constitute an important phase of their work. However, in adult care the trend toward preventive medicine is only gradually taking hold. In the hope of hastening this process, the simplicity and ease of preventive care for one of the major threats to adult health, coronary heart disease, will be described.

Based on our current knowledge of coronary risk factors, identification of high-risk individuals requires little cost and effort. Age, sex, family history, and pertinent habits such as cigarette smoking and exercise are simple historical items that can be obtained by paramedical personnel or self-administered questionnaires. Likewise, height and weight or simple observation to detect obesity and a blood-pressure measurement can be done by anyone in the office with minimal training. All that remains is an electrocardiogram and the drawing of a blood specimen for measuring cholesterol and glucose. A fasting blood specimen for triglyceride might be added, but there is some evidence suggesting that this adds little if the cholesterol is known.

Most authorities presently believe that persons with elevated levels of correctable risk factors should receive remedial therapy. As mentioned earlier, there is no safe cutoff point for each measure. The physician must form an overall impression of the patient's risk and act accordingly.

The remedial measures for the most part appear to be safe and consistent with good general health. Where appropriate, advice should be given to stop smoking, to eat less rich food in order to reduce weight and blood lipids, and to get more exercise without going to sudden extremes. Drugs that are apparently safe will lower blood pressure in most cases and will reduce lipid levels that do not respond sufficiently to diet.

The point that requires emphasis is that the detection and treatment of high coronary risk is simple and should be well within the scope of office medical practice. It would be naïve to assume that all high-risk patients will stop smoking, or eat less, or exercise more, if a doctor tells them to. Probably most will not. But some will, and it would be a shame if they were not given the opportunity and encouragement to lower their risk for a frequent, often fatal, disease.

CRITICAL READING OF THE MEDICAL LITERATURE

Most health-care professionals do not have enough time available for the careful reading and study of all the medical and scientific articles that come to their attention. It is important, however, to be able to evaluate critically reports and papers that can influence clinical decision or practice.

It is not intended, in this brief discussion, to cover all the errors and pitfalls that can occur in medical papers. Evaluating methods, observations, and interpretations in specialized fields such as surgery or biochemistry often requires knowledge and experience in the particular discipline.

An understanding of epidemiology does foster a critical approach to certain aspects of papers involving the study of populations or patient groups. The following discussion will focus primarily on some common problems and fallacies of an epidemiologic or statistical nature. The basic principles involved should already be familiar to the reader as they have been mentioned in previous chapters.

Need for an Adequate Control Group or Basis of Comparison

Many papers report findings apparently showing the benefits of a preventive or treatment measure, based on what appear to be good results, when the measure has been used on a study group. In viewing these "good results" the reader should always ask, *Compared to what?* This initial question will usually imply others such as, *Was there a control or comparison group? Who constituted the control group? Were they similar to the treated group in all important aspects other than the treatment?* The author should have provided clear and satisfying answers to these questions in the paper. If not, there is good reason to doubt the claimed benefits.

It might be found, for example, that 95 percent of those given a certain hypnotic drug reported the next day that they slept soundly. Although, at first glance, this in itself sounds like impressive evidence for the efficacy of the drug, we must know what percentage of similar but untreated persons would report sleeping soundly on the previous night. Furthermore, to rule out a placebo effect, we need to know what percentage, given an inactive "sleeping pill," would similarly report sound sleep.

The demonstration of harmful effects also requires a basis of comparison. It may be recalled from Chap. 7 that it was not sufficient to show that a large proportion of fatally injured pedestrians have high blood-alcohol levels to incriminate alcohol as a contributor to being struck and killed by a motor vehicle. It was also necessary to demonstrate that noninjured pedestrians, otherwise similar to those killed, had, on the average, *less* alcohol in their blood.

Requirement of Denominators for Statements Comparing Risks

Statements implying that a factor involves greater or less risk of a certain outcome are often made using only "numerator" data. The reader should "think epidemiologically" and remember that statements concerning risk should be based on *rates*, which require *denominators* as well as numerators. An example, again regarding motor-vehicle accidents, comes from a radio advertisement of a few years ago promoting the use of auto seat belts. A statement was made to the effect that 75 percent of all motor-vehicle fatalities occurred within 25 miles of home. The implication seemed to be that it was especially risky to drive on short trips close to home. However, note that motor-vehicle fatalities constitute only the numerator of a mortality rate, which needs also an appropriate denominator, such as passenger-miles. If, say, 95 percent of all passenger miles were driven within 25 miles of home, it could easily be shown that the *risk* of getting killed per passenger mile is *less* within 25 miles of home than it is farther away.

Failure to choose the appropriate denominator in drawing conclusions about risk is an easy error to fall into. One might note that the age distribution of a large series of 500 myocardial infarction cases observed at a particular institution was as shown in Table 13-1.

It would be tempting but erroneous to conclude on the basis of these data that the risk of myocardial infarction rises with age into the sixties and then falls sharply. Statements about risk at various ages must be related to the underlying population from which the cases are drawn. Incidence rates should be constructed by using the number of cases at each age as the numerator and the number of

Table 13-1   Hypothetical Age Distribution of Myocardial Infarction Cases

Age	Number of cases	Percent
20–29	10	2
30–39	40	8
40–49	75	15
50–59	125	25
60–69	175	35
70–79	50	10
80+	25	5
Total	500	100

persons at risk in the denominator. These will permit an appropriate comparison of risk at different ages. Fallacious inferences about risk, of the type illustrated here, are frequent and should be watched for.

Other Problems

A variety of special problems involving particular concepts, measurements, or study designs have been discussed in previous chapters. Examples are the possibility for spurious correlations due to uncontrolled variables, the need to distinguish statistical from biological significance (Chap. 11) and the likelihood of biased comparisons of survival when the starting point for follow-up is different in two groups (Chap. 10). Perhaps the reader's attention should again be called to the discussions in Chap. 3 on the limitations of medical observations, to the sections in Chaps. 4 through 10 concerning the conduct and interpretation of various types of studies, and to the interpretation of statistical associations as described in Chap. 11. In addition, much of the advice on conducting a study in Chap. 12 is also pertinent to evaluation the studies of others. Further discussion of problems and fallacies can be found in Ludwig and Collette (1971), Schor and Karten (1966), Hill (1971), and Huff (1954).

Although they are not solely epidemiologic concerns, some other general points deserve consideration in reading critically. These are discussed below.

Possibilities for Bias

The possibilities for biased comparisons are many. Misleading differences between groups may result from differences in the way they were selected, differences in the way data were collected from them, different follow-up durations, different criteria for judging outcome, and so on. The critical reader should try to think of these sources of bias and should note whether the author has taken them into account in his study methods or data analysis. Important potential biases should at least be mentioned in the Discussion section of a paper, if they could not be excluded.

Need for Adequate Information

It is important to determine whether the author has described his methods of selecting subjects, and of collecting and analyzing data in enough detail so that they can be evaluated and so that others can try to repeat the study or understand why their findings might differ. By close attention to these methods, the critical reader may also be able to determine whether the study was done with care or rather haphazardly.

Evidence of Objectivity

Some attempt should be made to determine whether the author appears to be objective or whether he is an advocate of a particular point of view. Is the presentation slanted toward a particular viewpoint? Would the author have published the paper if the opposite findings had been observed? Some knowledge of his previous work may be helpful in answering these questions.

One way that lack of objectivity may affect study results is through a selection process. Without intending to be misleading, an investigator may emphasize those observations which support his point of view and discard those that do not. Referring again to Fig. 11-1, page 152, which shows a moderate correlation between coronary heart disease mortality and per capita cigarette consumption in 44 states, note that the points for Utah, Arkansas, Kentucky, Indiana, and Connecticut fall along a straight line. If one wanted to show that the two variables had a nearly perfect correlation, one could prepare a graph showing these five states only. These five points would indeed present an impressive picture, if it were not mentioned that they were selected out of all the available data.

Selection for Publication

Viewing the medical literature as a whole, it is clear that positive findings are more apt to appear than negative findings. It must be remembered that positive findings may occur by chance where there is no relationship. Even when the authors are objective, chance positive findings are more apt to find their way into the literature than truly negative findings, at least until controversy makes negative findings just as important and interesting as positive findings.

REFERENCES

Dry, T. J., *Manual of Cardiology.* (Philadelphia: W. B. Saunders, 1943) pp. 1,2.

Hill, A. B., *Principles of Medical Statistics*, 9th ed. (London: Oxford University Press, 1971), Chaps. 21–23.

Huff, D., *How to Lie with Statistics.* (New York: W. W. Norton, 1954).

Ludwig, E. G., and J. C. Collette. 1971. Some misuses of health statistics. *J. Am. Med. Assoc.*, **216**:493–499.

Price, W. H. 1963. Gall-bladder dyspepsia. *Brit. Med. J.*, **2**:138–141.

Schor, S., and I. Karten. 1966. Statistical evaluation of medical journal manuscripts. *J. Am. Med. Assoc.*, **195**:1123–1128.

Weiss, N. S. 1972. Relation of high blood pressure to headache, epistaxis, and selected other symptoms: The United States health examination survey of adults. *New Engl. J. Med.*, **287**:631–633.

Chapter 14

Epidemiology, Medical Care, and the Health of the Community

Health and disease in the community are important concerns not only of medical and public health professionals but of the general public as well. To illustrate the important role of epidemiology in community health, two types of epidemiologic investigations will be described briefly—the time-honored investigation of infectious-disease epidemics and some recent efforts to detect unsuspected environmental hazards. Then, the limited effects of medical care on community health will be discussed. Screening for disease and other methods for increasing the beneficial effects of health care on the community will then be described.

Investigation of Epidemics of Infectious Disease

Until a few decades ago, epidemiology had focused primarily on the infectious diseases, which have been the major scourges of man-kind. Recently, in the more affluent nations, most infectious diseases have been brought under reasonably good control, and the leading causes of death and disability have become the noninfectious conditions. Thus, in these areas, many epidemiologists' attention has been directed toward chronic degenerative and neoplastic diseases. Other diseases or conditions of great interest and importance include physical trauma or accidents, mental illness, and congenital defects. Additional concerns that have recently engaged the epidemiologist are studies of medical care and health services, and studies that focus on general health status irrespective of the particular diseases responsible for departures from good health.

Despite a shifting emphasis in the more affluent nations, infectious diseases remain extremely important problems in the "less developed" parts of the world. Furthermore, dangerous infectious-disease outbreaks continue to occur in industrialized nations. Even though the principal causes of many of these diseases are fairly well understood, epidemiologists, health officers, other physicians and public-health nurses are still called upon to investigate specific disease outbreaks to determine the particular conditions or factors that are responsible.

Investigation of the variety of epidemics that might occur cannot be described by a single step-by-step "cookbook" approach. However, certain principles are followed sufficiently often to deserve at least a brief summary here. The interested reader should consult Anderson et al. (1962) for more details.

The typical field investigation of an epidemic involves, first, a study of the cases. Clinical examination and appropriate laboratory tests are needed to determine or verify the diagnosis. Once the disease is identified, knowledge of the usual sources of infection and common modes of spread for that disease will help point the investigation toward the most likely explanations of the epidemic. A convenient reference book that summarizes the important information for most infectious diseases is *Control of Communicable Diseases in Man*, published by the American Public Health Association (Benenson (ed.), 1970).

In addition to verifying the diagnosis, the patients are studied further, usually by interview. Their basic characteristics such as age, sex, and occupation should be determined, as should the onset and time course of the disease. Personal contacts at home, work, school, and other places, special events such as parties and trips, foods eaten, and exposures to other common vehicles are items that will frequently be inquired about, depending, of course, on the disease believed responsible for the outbreak. Particular emphasis should be placed on the time period when the patient was most probably infected. This period precedes the disease onset time by an interval equal to the usual incubation period for that disease.

The subsequent investigation will be guided by information gained from the known cases. For example, plotting the dates of disease onset graphically as in Figs. 5–7 (page 69), 5–8 (page 71), and 5–9 (page 72) will help determine if the epidemic had a point-source or involved person-to-person spread. Or, if the disease involves a gastrointestinal infection and several cases mention going to the same restaurant or party, further investigation of possible food contamination at the restaurant or party would be in order. Pursuing the party further, apparently well persons who also attended it might also be given appropriate laboratory tests to detect subclinical infection. Comparisons of what the infected and uninfected persons ate at the party will help determine which foods were contaminated. A good example of the simple analyses that are made to identify foods that serve as vehicles for infection is presented and discussed by Sartwell (1965).

Data analysis concerning possible causative factors for an epidemic will usually take the form either of an incidence study or a case-control study. In the former approach the incidence, or "attack" rates, of persons exposed to possible sources or vehicles are compared with those of persons not exposed. If the rates are much higher in the exposed, the source is highly suspect. In the case-control comparison, the suspect sources are those to which a much higher proportion of cases than controls were exposed.

It is hoped that investigation of the epidemic will reveal correctible problems. A major accomplishment would be the identification of infected persons who can continue to spread disease if not attended to, such as typhoid carriers working in restaurants or hospital employees with staphylococcal skin infections. The recognition of other factors leading to the spread of disease, such as improper food-handling practices, contaminated water supplies, or segments of the population who have not received the usual vaccinations, can also lead to effective control measures.

The Detection and Evaluation of Environmental Hazards

In recent years there has been considerable concern that we are poisoning ourselves with our technology. It is well known that our land, water, and air are being polluted by such substances as industrial wastes, exhaust products from burning fuels, trace metals, chemicals, pesticides, and radioactive materials. Furthermore, the population now ingests a variety of chemicals in such forms as preservatives and medicinal drugs.

What is less clear is the extent to which these substances affect human health. Epidemiologic studies can play an important role in the quantitative determination of the risks involved.

The usual investigations have employed standard epidemiologic methods to assess the relationship between specific substances, drugs, energy sources, or occupational exposures, and particular disease outcomes of interest. Examples are the Berlin, New Hampshire prevalence study of chronic respiratory disease in relation to air pollution and smoking, described in Chap. 6, the case-control study of thromboembolic disease in relation to oral contraceptives described in Chap. 7, and the cohort study of occupational exposure to x-ray described in Chap. 8. (For further examples, see Whittenberger, 1967, and Goldsmith, 1972).

These studies involve an assessment of environmental hazards that are *already under suspicion.* The proliferation of new chemicals and energy sources to which we are exposed has led to serious concern that there are many hazards that we are not aware of. Sometimes, unsuspected hazards come to light only after considerable damage has been done. A recent dramatic example involved the drug thalidomide which, when given as a tranquilizer to pregnant women, resulted in the birth of thousands of seriously deformed babies. Other classical cases were the occurrence of retrolental fibroplasia in premature infants who received oxygen therapy, and the development of bone cancers in radium-dial painters.

As a result of concern for the unsuspected, epidemiologists

have begun to work in a new area of research, sometimes called *monitoring*. The purpose of monitoring is to detect unsuspected adverse or undesired effects of components of the environment as soon as possible after these effects appear, and thus provide an "early warning system." Because broad areas are to be covered, this type of investigation usually involves initially a search for hypotheses. Suspicious relationships can then be subjected to more intensive study.

Much of the experience to date in monitoring environmental hazards has been gained from monitoring adverse reactions to medicinal drugs (Report of the International Conference on Adverse Reactions Reporting System, 1971). Despite careful testing of drugs before they are marketed, many drug reactions do not become recognized until the drug has been extensively used by large numbers of patients. Monitoring of drug reactions will be used to illustrate some of the methods to be described.

A number of methods or systems of monitoring are available. These have been tried with varying degrees of success. They involve the assembly and analysis of data on morbid events, usually, but not always, in relation to various exposures.

Spontaneous Reporting Systems   Many hypotheses come from the observation by individual physicians of patients who develop what seems to be an adverse reaction to a drug. Ordinarily, if he is sufficiently concerned, the physician might report this to the drug manufacturer or publish a letter or brief case report in a medical journal.

Programs known as spontaneous reporting systems have been established to encourage physicians to send such reports to a central agency or clearing house where they can be assembled and evaluated. Examples are the reporting programs that have been set up by the Food and Drug Administration in the United States and the Committee on Safety of Drugs in the United Kingdom.

While some useful information has been obtained at low cost from spontaneous reports, certain deficiencies are apparent. Despite promotional efforts to get physicians to respond, the number of reports submitted and the amount of information contained in each report have often been disappointing. Furthermore, it is very difficult for the physician to determine the cause of a serious untoward event in a single patient. While it could be an adverse effect of a drug, it could also be a worsening or complication of the disease being treated, or even the result of a different disease that has developed independently. Physicians tend to recognize and interpret as drug reactions events that they are familiar with in that regard, such as skin rash following penicillin therapy or aplastic anemia following chloramphenicol; they tend not to report unsuspected relationships. Finally, the lack of any "denominator" or "population-at-risk" information makes it difficult to determine whether the reaction might be rare or relatively common.

Changes in Disease Frequency If a population is being exposed to a new environmental hazard or to increased levels of an old hazard, suspicion can be aroused by monitoring disease frequency. Populations or special subgroups may be kept under systematic surveillance to determine time trends in incidence, prevalence, or mortality from any or all diseases. A good example is the monitoring of congenital malformations in newborn infants. The prevalence of various malformations among newborn infants in several cooperating hospitals can be recorded on a monthly basis. If the occurrence of one or more malformations shows a distinct increase beyond the fluctuations usually noted due to chance or seasonal variations, then an inquiry into prenatal exposures might be initiated, much as one would investigate an epidemic of infectious disease (Hook, 1972).

Although probably less accurate than special programs to monitor disease frequency, the surveillance of vital statistics can also provide useful information about changes in disease frequency. Increases in mortality rates in communities or increases in congenital malformations reported on birth certificates can provide useful clues that something is happening in the environment.

Intensive Surveillance of Both Exposures and Disease Procedures can be established to collect extensive information concerning both exposures and disease frequency. In this way a variety of exposure/disease relationships can be explored to look for unsuspected relationships and to develop quantitative information about known relationships. An example of this type of program is the

Community Health and Environmental Surveillance System (CHESS) of the Environmental Protection Agency, in which several components of air pollution and several measures of health and disease are measured in selected communities (Riggan et al., 1972). Examples in drug-reaction monitoring are the Boston Collaborative Drug Surveillance Program (Jick et al., 1970) which collects and analyzes data about drug administration and untoward events from several hospitals, and the Kaiser-Permanente Drug-Reaction Monitoring System, which emphasizes drug use and drug reactions in outpatients (Friedman et al., 1971).

Limited Effects of Medical Care—Historical Perspective

With the impressive technical advances in medical care that have become available in recent decades, it is easy to forget that the quality and quantity of medical care have only a limited influence on community health. That medical care is not the only determinant of health is well illustrated by the observed long-term time trends in mortality from certain diseases. As will be shown, these trends appear to bear little relationship to changes in medical care.

One example is the marked decline in mortality from tuberculosis in the United States during the twentieth century (Fig. 14-1). As pointed out by Winkelstein (1972), the only treatment available at the beginning of this century was rest therapy in sanatoriums, accessible only to the wealthy. This was made available to all economic classes in the 1930's, and during the same decade, collapse therapy was introduced. Chemotherapy became widely available in the 1950's. Fig. 14-1 shows that the downward trend in mortality was clearly evident before these new therapies were widely applied. Winkelstein also cited data from a study by Terris (1948) showing that the isolation of cases in treatment facilities was probably not a major determinant of tuberculosis mortality. Thus, even though therapy and isolation of cases may have accentuated the decline shown in Fig. 14-1, other important factors must have been operating.

Other diseases have also shown major secular changes that are difficult to attribute to the benefits of medical care. For example, McKeown and Lowe (1966) presented a graphic picture of the

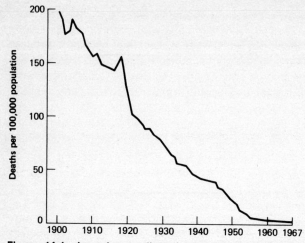

Figure 14-1 Annual age-adjusted tuberculosis death rates per 100,000 population, death registration states of the United States, 1900–1967. (Adjusted to the age distribution of the U.S. population in 1940.) *(Reproduced, by permission, from Winkelstein, 1972.)*

decline in mortality from whooping cough in English children, similar to that shown for tuberculosis in Fig. 14-1. Mortality declined rather steadily from about 1,400 deaths per million per year in 1870 to a negligible number in the 1960's. Relevant medical landmarks during this decline were the identification of the causative organism in 1906, sulfonamide and antibiotic therapy, beginning in 1939, and the general availability of immunization beginning in 1952. By the time drug therapy and immunization became available, the whooping cough mortality rate was only a small fraction of what it had been in the late nineteenth century, when it was a very important cause of death.

The rather striking time trends over the last few decades in lung cancer and stomach cancer mortality rates (see Fig. 5-10, page 75) are also largely independent of the effects of medical care. To date, medical, surgical, and radiation therapy cannot save the lives of the vast majority of victims of these two malignancies.

It is obvious from these examples and from the usual incurability of the degenerative and neoplastic diseases that constitute most of our leading causes of death and disability, that if we are to bring these conditions under control and improve the health and longevity of the population, we cannot rely solely on increasing the availability of medical care as we know it today. More important will be to improve our understanding of the environmental and social factors which foster these diseases and, using this knowledge, to apply effective preventive measures.

Two Aspects of Disease Prevention

One approach to disease prevention is through medical care of individual patients. As an example of this approach, a simple method for preventing coronary heart disease, to be used in the clinic or physician's office, was described in Chap. 13. It involved, first, detecting individuals who are at high risk of developing the disease, and secondly, attempting to reduce their risk by changing their dietary and other habits and judiciously prescribing drugs, when indicated.

The second avenue of disease prevention does not focus on the individual. Rather, it involves large-scale social and environmental changes, such as improving housing conditions, requiring pasteurization of all milk sold commercially, or adding fluoride to community water supplies. For coronary heart disease, possible preventive approaches on this scale might include changing food processing to decrease the amount of saturated fat and cholesterol in animal food products, discouraging cigarette smoking by increased taxes or by other forms of persuasion well known to the advertising industry, or discovering the harmful agents in tobacco smoke and removing them, or banning automobiles from certain areas so as to force many people to walk or ride bicycles. These measures are listed here as examples of efforts that might be considered, not as proven practical approaches to the problem of coronary heart disease.

Because many people do not go to doctors routinely and because many others who do go either do not follow medical advice or find it extremely difficult to break pleasurable habits, one is forced into a rather pessimistic view about the impact that office preventive medicine can have on the health of the general population. Even special intensive programs to change patient behavior have not proven to have as much long-term effect as has been hoped. For example, a variety of innovative methods have been tried to help people stop smoking cigarettes. Despite high initial success rates, follow-up one year later usually reveals that only about one-fifth of those originally treated still refrain from smoking.

The health-care professional must do what he can to help his patients. Certainly a success rate of one out of five is better than nothing. Nevertheless, since medical care often has so little impact on major health problems of the community, many believe that only large-scale social and environmental changes will be effective.

The Physician's Limited View of Disease in the Community

One reason that medical care has less influence than one might expect is that much disease never comes to the attention of medical personnel. Using prevalence survey data obtained in Great Britain and the United States, White, Williams, and Greenberg (1961) showed how illness in the community gets filtered to various physicians and institutions in the medical-care system. As shown in Fig. 14-2, of 1,000 adults in the community, 750 report one or more illnesses each month. One-third of those with illnesses, or 250, consult a physician. Only 9, or 1.2 percent of the ill are admitted to a hospital, and only 5, or 0.7 percent, are referred to another physician. Particularly striking from the viewpoint of medical education is the fact that only one of these patients is seen at a university medical center.

Not only do just a portion of the sick get seen medically, but each medical specialty and medical setting attracts a selected group of patients out of all those seen. For example, in the outpatient clinic one is especially apt to encounter patients with mild acute and chronic illness and patients with symptoms for which no organic basis can be found. In the hospital, patients are, on the average, much more seriously ill with diseases that are farther advanced. As pointed out by White et al., "Each practitioner or administrator sees a biased sample of medical care problems presented to him; rarely has any individual, specialty or institution a broad appreciation of the ecology of medical care that enables unique and frequently

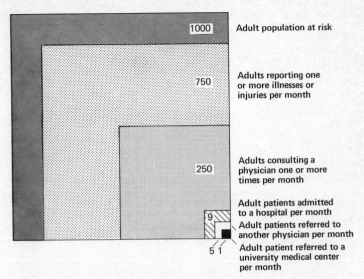

Figure 14-2 Monthly prevalence estimates of illness in the community and the roles of physicians, hospitals, and University Medical Centers in the provision of medical care (adults 16 years of age and over). *(Reproduced, by permission, from White, Williams, and Greenberg, 1961.)*

isolated contributions to be seen in relation to those of others and to the over-all needs of the community."

Efforts to Bring More Disease to Medical Attention: Screening

In the hope of increasing the impact of current medical knowledge and technology on disease in the community, medical and public health facilities have established *screening* programs to detect persons with early, mild, and asymptomatic disease.

As stated by Thorner and Remein (1961), "The basic purpose of screening for disease detection is to separate from a large group of apparently well persons those who have a high probability of having the disease under study, so that they may be given a diagnostic workup and, if diseased, brought to treatment." Since screening tests are designed to be applicable to large population groups, they must be simple, rapid and inexpensive. As a result, they are generally less accurate and definitive than the examinations and tests used by physicians to arrive at a final diagnosis.

Screening is carried out in the belief that the detection of disease in an early or asymptomatic stage will lead to appropriate treatment which, in turn, will lead to less disability and/or mortality from the disease. After an initial period of enthusiasm in some quarters, considerable skepticism developed concerning the benefits of screening, based on doubts as to whether it would really lead to favorable modifications in the course of disease.

Critics pointed out that many persons with diseases discovered by screening did not receive adequate or appropriate treatment afterward. Or, even if the accepted treatment is given for some diseases detected by screening, such as mild maturity-onset diabetes mellitus, it has not been shown that persons so treated live happier, healthier, or longer lives. Also, persons correctly or incorrectly labeled as having a disease would be caused considerable worry and anxiety, often to no good purpose. Furthermore, careful analysis showed that apparently good results of screening could be misleading, due to self-selection for screening of those persons who take better care of themselves, or due to fallacies such as that pointed out in Chap. 10, page 148, wherein persons would *seem* to survive longer merely because the diagnosis was made earlier. Even ethical questions have been raised (McKeown, 1968) since in contrast to traditional medical care which is sought by the patient, disease detection by screening is initiated by medical or public health professionals, who, therefore, are under special obligation to make sure that screening does more good than harm.

Thus, evaluation of screening programs requires carefully controlled experimental studies in which relevant disease outcomes are measured in a group receiving screening and compared to outcomes measured similarly in a comparable unscreened group. Any benefits found for screening programs should be compared to costs involved (McKeown and Knox, 1968; Wilson, 1968; Cochrane and Holland, 1971). Although it is more an evaluation of periodic comprehensive health checkups than of screening per se, the Kaiser-Permanente Multiphasic Health Checkup Evaluation Study, described in Chap. 9, illustrates the approach that is needed if screening programs are to prove their merits. Other examples of well-controlled evaluations of screening or disease-detection methods are the study of breast cancer screening by the Health Insurance Plan of New York (Shapiro, Strax, and Venet, 1971) and the study of lung cancer screening by Brett (1971).

A generally accepted principle is that screening should only be done if it can be integrated with the medical-care program where it is carried out. In practice this means not only that adequate treatment, care, and follow-up be available for those who screen positive, but that the screening test results must be acceptable to the practicing physicians in the area. The characteristics of screening tests that relate to accuracy and acceptability will be discussed briefly.

Sensitivity and specificity, two measures of the accuracy of diagnostic tests, were defined in Chap. 13, page 192. These measures are also important features of screening tests. The relationship of a screening test to the final accurate diagnosis is conveniently shown in a fourfold table (see Table 14-1). In the table, a represents persons with the disease who are correctly labeled by the screening test. Persons denoted by b are *false positives*, since the test is positive but they do not have the disease. The letter d denotes persons free of disease who are correctly labeled by the test. The letter c represents *false negatives*, persons with the disease for whom the test is negative.

Sensitivity, the proportion of true positives that are labeled as positive, is thus $a/(a + c)$. Specificity, the proportion of true negatives that are labeled as negative is $d/(b + d)$. Both of these measures are important, since the test should detect as much disease as possible while avoiding false labeling. False negatives,

Table 14-1   Relationship of Screening-Test Results to the Final Accurate Diagnosis

| Screening test | Final diagnosis | | Total |
	Disease present	Disease absent	
Positive	a	b	$a + b$
Negative	c	d	$c + d$
Total	$a + c$	$b + d$	$a + b + c + d$

persons with undetected disease, may be deprived of valuable therapy. False positives, persons incorrectly labeled as diseased, are subject to needless worry and expensive diagnostic evaluations until their freedom from the disease is established. With all quantitative screening tests, the level above or below which a person is called positive will affect the sensitivity and specificity. Modifying this cutoff level to improve one of these characteristics will adversely affect the other.

Physicians evaluating patients who have been screened are especially sensitive to another measure, $a/(a + b)$, the proportion of positive tests that are true positives. Since physicians are usually asked to evaluate only the positive screenees, they understandably become irritated and critical of the screening program when most of their follow-up diagnostic evaluations turn out to be negative.

If the disease is infrequent in the population—and most chronic diseases are—even a screening test with a high degree of specificity will yield positives of which a large percentage turn out to be false. Thorner and Remein (1961) showed an example of a population of 10,000 with an assumed prevalence of diabetes mellitus of 1.5 percent, screened with a random blood glucose (not drawn at any particular time in relation to eating). Using a cutoff point of 130 mg percent, the test has been shown previously to have a sensitivity of 44.3 percent and a high specificity of 99.0 percent. The results are shown in Table 14-2. Note, that of the 164 positives, 98, or 60 percent, turn out to be false positives.

If, in order to decrease the number of false positives, the screening level is raised to 180 mg percent, the specificity will now

Table 14-2   Results of Screening for Diabetes Mellitus in a Population of 10,000*

Screening test	Final Diagnosis		Total
	Diabetic	Not diabetic	
Positive	66	98	164
Negative	84	9,752	9,836
Total	150	9,850	10,000

*In this population the disease prevalence is 1.5%, and the sensitivity and specificity of the test are 44.3% and 99.0%, respectively.
Source: Data from Thorner and Remein (1961).

be 99.8 percent. The test will now yield only 54 positives, of whom only 20, or 37 percent, are false positive. However, there is a marked decrease in sensitivity. Only 34 of the 150 diabetics will be detected.

If the disease prevalence is higher, a larger proportion of positives will be true positives. One strategy for increasing the prevalence of disease in the population screened is to restrict screening to high-risk individuals. For example, screening for diabetes by measuring blood sugar may be carried out only among persons who are obese or who have a family history of the disease.

Broadening the Concept of Screening

Although formal screening programs were initially directed primarily at the early detection of single specific diseases, the screening concept has expanded in recent years to encompass *screening for high risk* and *multiphasic screening.*

Screening for High Risk   As more emphasis is being placed on disease prevention, community programs for disease control may well include screening programs to detect persons at high risk of developing disease. In this way, preventive measures can be applied before the disease occurs. For example, pilot programs are now underway in industry and communities to identify persons with coronary risk factors such as high serum-cholesterol and blood-pressure levels, so that myocardial infarction and other manifestations of coronary heart disease can be prevented. The long-term effects of these programs need to be evaluated.

Before setting up such a program it is necessary, as with screening for frank disease, to make sure that suitable care and follow-up will be available for positive screenees. That is, the screening must fit in with the local medical care program so that something more than patient anxiety will result.

Multiphasic Screening   It is more efficient to screen for a variety of diseases at one time than to carry out separate screening programs for single diseases. Fostered by the development of automated testing procedures, *multiphasic* screening programs are becoming widespread.

Multiphasic screening or multiphasic health testing is being viewed increasingly as having greater utility than just in the detection of asymptomatic disease (Thorner, 1969). It has been shown to be an efficient and economical component of periodic health check-ups for patients both with and without known disease. Used in this way, multiphasic screening of high quality appears to be acceptable to both physicians and patients, and it conserves physician time and other medical-care resources (Collen, 1971).

Multiphasic health testing is also seen now as an important component of a new mode of entry of patients into medical care. With the trend toward prepayment or government payment for medical care, the traditional economic barrier, the fee for service, is disappearing. To prevent a resultant overloading of the medical-care system and to assure appropriate allocation of physician time to the care of the sick, Garfield (1970) has proposed a new system of organization for medical care. He suggested that patients not acutely ill enter the system in a way that would utilize multiphasic health testing to help determine the nature of the problem and the appropriate facility to which the patient should be referred.

Evaluating a Changing Health-Care System

We are living in a period of great change in health care. Spurred by technological and socioeconomic advances, many old methods are being questioned or discarded and new approaches are being introduced.

Innovations can and should be evaluated by well-controlled experiments, whenever possible. Where particular circumstances or meager resources prohibit rigorous experiments, less-formal evaluations such as before/after comparisons can be conducted. However, careful attention should then be paid to extraneous influences and biasing factors that may affect the apparent outcomes of the innovation.

A few of the health care issues of current interest are modes of payment for services, the use of nurses and other paramedical personnel for tasks traditionally performed by physicians, the content and frequency of health checkups and community screening programs, control of drug overuse and abuse, and provision of optimal care for persons living in inner cities and remote rural areas. Defining and describing these problems, and identifying and evaluating possible solutions all involve studies of health-related characteristics, events, and outcomes in groups of people.

Whether these studies are labeled as "epidemiology," or "medical-care research," or "health-services research" makes little difference. What is important is that we be guided by careful observations and wise judgment to make necessary improvements while preserving the many good methods and approaches that we now have.

REFERENCES

Anderson, G. W., M. G. Arnstein, and M. R. Lester, *Communicable Disease Control: A Volume for the Public Health Worker*, 4th ed. (New York: Macmillan, 1962) Chap. 10.

Benenson, A. S. (Ed.), *Control of Communicable Diseases in Man.* 11th ed. (New York: American Public Health Association, 1970).

Brett, G. Z. 1968. The value of lung cancer detection by six monthly chest radiographs. *Thorax*, **23**:414–420.

Cochrane, A. L., and W. W. Holland. 1971. Validation of screening procedures. *Brit. Med. Bull.*, **27**:3–8.

Collen, M. F. 1971. Guidelines for multiphasic health checkups. *Arch. Intern. Med.*, **127**:99–100.

Friedman, G. D., M. F. Collen, L. E. Harris, E. E. Van Brunt, and L. S. Davis. 1971. Experience in monitoring drug reactions in outpatients: The Kaiser-Permanente Drug Monitoring System. *J. Am. Med. Assoc.*, **217**:567–572.

Garfield, S. R. 1970. The delivery of medical care. *Sci. Am.*, **222**:15–23.

Goldsmith, J. R., Statistical Problems and Strategies in Environmental Epidemiology. *Proceedings of the Sixth Berkeley Symposium on Mathematical Statistics and Probability. vol. VI Effects of Pollution on Health.* (Berkeley: University of California Press, 1972), pp. 1–28.

Hook, E. B., Monitoring Human Birth Defects, Methods and Strategies. *Proceedings of the Sixth Berkeley Symposium on Mathematical Statistics and Probability. vol. VI Effects of Pollution on Health.* (Berkeley: University of California Press, 1972), pp. 355–366.

Jick, H., O. S. Miettinen, S. Shapiro, G. P. Lewis, V. Siskind, and D. Slone. 1970. Comprehensive drug surveillance. *J. Am. Med. Assoc.*, **213**:1455–1460.

McKeown, T.: Validation of Screening Procedures, in *Screening in Medicine: Reviewing the Evidence: A Collection of Essays.* (London: Oxford University Press, 1968), pp. 1–13.

McKeown, T., and E. G. Knox, The Framework Required for Validation of Prescriptive Screening, in *Screening in Medicine: Reviewing the Evidence: A Collection of Essays.* (London: Oxford University Press, 1968), pp. 159–173.

McKeown, T., and C. R. Lowe: *An Introduction to Social Medicine.* (Philadelphia: F. A. Davis, 1966), pp. 86–87.

Report of the International Conference on Adverse Reactions Reporting Systems. National Academy of Sciences, Washington, D.C. 1971.

Riggan, W. B., D. I. Hammer, J. F. Finklea, V. Hasselblad, C. R. Sharp, R. M. Burton, and C. M. Shy, CHESS, A Community Health and Environmental Surveillance System. *Proceedings of the Sixth Berkeley Symposium on Mathematical Statistics and Probability. vol. VI Effects of Pollution on Health.* (Berkeley: University of California Press, 1972), pp. 111–123.

Sartwell, P. E. (ed.), *Maxcy-Rosenow Preventive Medicine and Public Health*, 9th ed. (New York: Appleton-Century-Crofts, 1965), pp. 16–19.

Shapiro, S., P. Strax, and L. Venet. 1971. Periodic breast cancer screening in reducing mortality from breast cancer. *J. Am. Med. Assoc.*, **215**:1777–1785.

Terris, M. 1948. Relation of economic status to tuberculosis mortality by age and sex. *Am. J. Public Health*, **38**:1061–1070.

Thorner, R. M. 1969. Whither multiphasic screening? *New Engl. J. Med.*, **280**:1037–1042.

Thorner, R. M. and Q. R. Remein, *Principles and Procedures in the Evaluation of Screening for Disease.* U.S. Department of Health, Education, and Welfare. Public Health Monograph no. 67, 1961.

White, K. L., T. F. Williams, B. G. Greenberg. 1961. The ecology of medical care. *New Engl. J. Med.*, **265**:885–892.

Whittenberger, J. L., The physical and chemical environment, in *Preventive Medicine*, edited by D. W. Clark, B. MacMahon, (Boston: Little, Brown, 1967), pp. 630–638.

Wilson, J. M. G. November 1968.: The evaluation of the worth of early disease detection. *J. Roy. Coll. Gen. Pract., Suppl.*, **2**:48–57.

Winkelstein, W., Jr. 1972. Epidemiological considerations underlying the allocation of health and disease care resources. *Intern. J. Epidemiology*, **1**:69–74.

Index